MEDIA ACCLAIM

For everyday disorders the book holds sheaves of information... with names and properties of a hundred different cures given it can serve like an instant dictionary which could pinpoint a remedy for any illness.

— TIMES OF INDIA

From acidity to warts, from hydrocephalus to spermatorrhoea, all possible ailments have been covered... and cure for every disease is prescribed.

— THE MAIL

ABOUT THE AUTHOR

Dr. Yudhvir Singh is regarded as the father of Homoeopathy in Delhi. He was instrumental in establishing the Homoeopathic College and Hospital in Delhi and the Trust functioning under him runs over a dozen hospitals and dispensaries in the city. The present book is already a bestseller in its Hindi edition, having been published in hardcover as well as paperback.

For more books and updates:

HOMOEOPATHIC CURE FOR COMMON DISEASES

DR. YUDHVIR SINGH

Orient Paperbacks
DELHI | MUMBAI

Disclaimer: The information included in this book is general in nature and for reference and guidance only. It is not a substitute for medical advice and the readers are urged to consult their doctor before taking decisions which are medical in nature.

Homoeopathic Cure for Common Diseases

1st Published 1980
This Printing 2023

Published by:
Orient Paperbacks
(A division of Vision Books Pvt. Ltd.)
5A/8 Ansari Road, 1st Floor
Daryaganj, New Delhi-110 002
www.orientpaperbacks.in

Cover design by A.R. Designz

Print ISBN: 9788122200171
eISBN: 9788122206791

Printed and bound at TACT, New Delhi

CONTENTS

Part III

CHARACTERISTICS OF SOME IMPORTANT MEDICINES

INTRODUCTION

This book by an experienced Homoeopath of Delhi prescribes appropriate medicines for nearly all common and some chronic diseases, according to specific symptoms. It is a complete handbook on the subject and is of the use to doctors as well. The author who is no more, had 50 years of vast experience in Homoeopathic treatment.

PREFACE

It was some time in 1967-68 that a Hindi book named *Pariwar Chikitsa*, written by me, was published. The book commanded a good sale and during the last ten years, several editions of it have been published, including two low-priced paperback editions. Shri Vishwa Nath of Orient Paperbacks, on whose persuasion I had written the Hindi book, asked me to write one in English for the benefit of non-Hindi readers. Thus, this Homoeopathic guide in English is in your hands.

I have been practising Homoeopathy for the last 60 years, and I have tried my best to give the benefit of my experience to those who are desirous of treating ordinary day-to-day ailments of theirs and their kith and kin.

In India, as well as in foreign countries, there are thousands of laymen who take to such treatment themselves. Thus the diseases are nipped in the bud and a lot of trouble, anxiety, expenditure and inconvenience is avoided. Of course, in serious cases professionals are consulted.

But before taking the help of this book for treating any disease, I shall request my readers to carefully go through the first few pages in which I have tried to explain the principles of

Homoeopathy and have given some necessary instructions about the use of Homoeopathic medicines.

Though there are more than a thousand medicines in Homoeopathy, a family chest containing about a hundred medicines will serve the purpose of a layman for treating his and his family members' general ailments.

I may repeat my request that the introductory chapter must be thoroughly read and understood before taking a case in hand.

I once again thank Shri Vishwa Nath for persuading me to write this book.

— Yudhvir Singh

I

HOMOEOPATHY

1

THE BASIC PRINCIPLE

"LIKE CURES LIKE"

Though everyone knows something about Homoeopathy, people don't normally know enough about it and even some well educated persons have misunderstandings about this science. It is sometimes claimed that there is mention of such a science in ancient Ayurveda where they have mentioned the concept of *viparita arthakari chikitsa* (the medical cures that have an opposite effect), yet the present science of Homoeopathy is the discovery of the German physician Dr. Christian Friedrich Samuel Hahnemann, who was born on 10 April 1755 and breathed his last in 1843.

Dr. Hahnemann was born in the poor family of a painter of earthen pots at Meissen in the Saxony State of Germany. A mastermind as he was, he succeeded in obtaining the highest degree of M.D. when he was only 24. He was appointed Civil Surgeon in the Dresden Hospital. After some time he started private practice near Leipzig, but he was not satisfied with the medical science prevailing at that time and its methods of treatment.

It was in 1790 that an incident resulted in the discovery of Homoeopathy by him. Dr. Hahnemann while translating an

English *A Treatise on the Materia Medica* into German came across the description of Cinchona, a plant from which Quinine and its other compounds are derived.

It was claimed that Cinchona is the surest remedy of malarial fever. Dr. Hahnemann also knew that, but it was also mentioned therein that indiscriminate use of Cinchona produces symptoms similar to malaria. This point struck Dr. Hahnemann and to test the statement he used a decoction of Cinchona in large doses which produced symptoms of malarial fever in him. He began to think whether all the medicines in small doses cured the diseases or symptoms which they produced when taken in large doses. For six years he made experiments with about 300 medicines and in 1796 he confirmed and published that

> A medicine in minimum doses cures all such symptoms or diseases which it is capable of producing in a healthy person when taken in large doses.

"Like cures like'" (or *Similia Similibus Curantur*) is the basic principle of Homoeopathy. As soon as it was published, a revolution took place in the medical world. In 1810 he published his famous work *Organon of Medicine,* which is termed as the Bible of Homoeopathy and clearly and logically explains the above principle.

Now, Dr. Hahnemann began to practise medicine according to the newly discovered principle of "Like Cures Like." He was immensely successful in curing many so called chronic and incurable diseases. Many physicians started working on the lines suggested by him but quite a few became envious and tried to defame and discourage him. Thus came ups and downs in Dr. Hahnemann's career but he remained strong in his conviction. During the last years of his life he had a roaring practice in Paris.

As explained above, according to Homoeopathy, the curative power of a medicine depends upon its capacity to produce ailments or disease symptoms. For example, ARSENIC produces diarrhoea, vomiting, extreme prostration, burning, unquenchable thirst, anguish. If these very symptoms occur in a patient without taking ARSENIC, they shall be cured by giving him ARSENIC, but in very minute doses.

2

THE SECOND PRINCIPLE

MINIMISE THE DOSE TO INCREASE ITS CURING POWER

This brings us to the second great principle of Homoeopathy — *Minima Minimus*, smaller the dose, better the result.

To minimise the dose Dr. Hahnemann mixed the medicine with non-medicinal substances such as alcohol, distilled water or sugar of milk. By a special procedure not only the dose was minimised but it was also dynamised, i.e. as the molecules of the medicine were divided and subdivided, their curative power was increased. Though it was difficult to be explained in the days of Hahnemann, now it can be easily explained in accordance with the atomic theory. Hence the minimised doses, though termed dilutions in the early stages, were named as Potencies later on.

These Potencies are of two types: x Potency and c Potency. x Potencies are prepared by mixing well one part of the original medicine with 9 parts of Vehicle, i.e., alcohol or distilled water or sugar of milk in cases of solid drugs. Similarly, c Potencies are prepared by mixing one part of the original medicine with 99 parts of Vehicle.

A Potency prepared in this manner is called 1x or 1c. One part of it is again mixed, according to the given method, with 9 or 99 parts of Vehicle to obtain 2x or 2c — and this process is repeated to give up to 3, 4, 6, 15, 30, 200, 500, 1000 and 100000 Potencies. The higher the Potency the greater its dynamic power to cure.

Ordinarily x is always mentioned against the name of the drug such as ACONITE 1x, ACONITE 6x or 30x but c is not mentioned. ACONITE 30 means ACONITE 30c. 1000 is often mentioned as 1M, 10000 as 10M, 100000 as CM. The original medicine is called Mother Tincture which is indicated by the Greek alphabet θ (theta). As already mentioned, solid mother drugs are mixed with sugar of milk and grinded well in pestle and mortar according to prescribed procedure. This process of grinding is called triturating and the powder potencies are called triturations such as ARSENIC 3x TRIT., BARYTA CARB 6x TRIT., or CALCAREA PHOS 12x TRIT.

3

HOMOEOPATHY TREATS THE PATIENT, NOT THE DISEASE

The *Materia Medica* of Homoeopathy is nothing but the proving of the medicines on healthy bodies, i.e., the symptoms which a medicine produces in a healthy body when taken in physiological doses. Therefore, in Homoeopathy the name of a disease is not at all necessary to select the right medicine. *Homoeopathy treats the patient not the disease,* unlike other systems of medicine where diseases are treated. In fact, the so called any one disease manifests so many various symptoms that no one medicine can be prescribed for it.

For ages, we have been accustomed to treating diseases by names. We have also prescribed medicines according to names of diseases but have mentioned different symptoms of different medicines in the same disease. The nomenclature of diseases are according to some prominent part of the effected body or some prominent symptoms. For example, if our lungs are effected and congested, we call it Pneumonia; if there is chill and fever we call it Malaria. If there is pain in the heart we call it Angina, and so on. But it should be clear that even in one disease, for example, in Pneumonia some patients are restless with high fever and great thirst, but others have no thirst and no restlessness but would like to lie down silently. Some will not be able to lie on the left side, while others will feel uncomfortable by lying on the right side. In Malaria, too there are so many different symptoms varying from patient to patient. Homoeopathy depends much on these different symptoms. A patient craves for cold water during fever, the other is thirstless, another feels better by moving about and still another is worse by slightest motion.

Therefore, to select the right Homoeopathic remedy, we have to note the location of the disease, i.e., the part affected, the sensations of the patient and aggravation and ameliorations of the troubles.

To select the right remedy, therefore, we should carefully note all the symptoms in a patient. We should note what he says as well as what his relatives nursing him, say. We should then find which medicine in the Materia Medica produces all these symptoms, or at least a majority of important symptoms. If we succeed by careful comparison in finding out a similar medicine, the minutest doses of the same will cure the patient.

4

DISEASES: ACUTE AND CHRONIC

In Homoeopathy diseases are Acute or Chronic. Acute diseases or conditions are short and sharp, and the whole body is not necessarily affected. In Chronic conditions the body's vital force gets disturbed to their depths and the disease keeps recurring. Their treatment should be left entirely to the doctor.

Every chronic disease often begins as an acute one. Acute diseases are of short duration, i.e., they begin and end within days or weeks, such as cholera, malaria, fever, cold, catarrh, measles, etc. Chronic diseases are those whose duration extends to months and years, such as asthma, cancer, T.B., piles, etc.

In acute diseases symptoms appear, increase and either end in cure or in death. In such diseases medicines are given frequently — even at intervals of 5-10-15 minutes, according to the severity of symptoms. In chronic diseases Homoeopathic medicines are often repeated weekly or monthly or even at longer intervals.

5

BUILD A SYMPTOM PICTURE TO CURE THE DISEASE

In Homoeopathy we do not prescribe for a disease or a single symptom but we take into account all the symptoms of the patient. We compare them with the symptoms or characteristics of suggested medicines and then prescribe one single medicine for the totality of the symptoms.

Symptoms are physical as well as mental. Physical symptoms include temperature, pulse, variations in behaviour, excretions from the body like stools, urine, sweat, vomit, phlegm, etc. The time when the disease is aggravated or ameliorated and its exact locations on the body have to be carefully noted. These should be noted in as much detail as possible.

One should try to build a complete symptom picture of the patient, starting from the head downwards, in a systematic and orderly way.

Great importance is attached to mental symptoms. These include the patient's appetites, cravings, feelings of anxiety, apathy, anger, etc., his dreams, and also his aversions. One should then compare these symptoms with the characteristics of medicines and select whichever is closest. This should not be done in a hurry.

It should now be clear that in Homoeopathy every patient is treated individually according to the symptoms of his ailments, and if carefully selected remedies are administered in the initial stages, many chronic and serious diseases can be avoided. The remedy thus selected acts upon the Vital Force and gives it the right guidance. It is this Vital Force that eradicates the morbid symptoms in totality and restores the patient to normal health.

I would like to quote a few instances from my own experience to impress upon the readers the importance of mental symptoms. A female patient about 50 years of age had developed cancer in her breasts and one breast was removed in the hospital. After some time she developed a small tumour in the other breast and came to me for treatment. One of her mental symptoms helped me to select the right remedy for her cancer. She was afraid of being alone but at the same time was depressed, felt timid and averse to society. This particular condition indicated CONIUM which was given in 1000 potency and this saved the removal of the other breast. She has been well for the last 7-8 years. The tumour still exists though reduced to great extent and without any pain whatsoever.

Another instance of a patient at Ferozepur jail is as follows. It was in the beginning of 1945 that a Muslim Asst. Superintendent was transferred to this jail from another jail. He consulted me for his bleeding piles. He had become very anaemic and had grown weak and emaciated. I gave him medicine for 3-4 days but there was no relief. He came to me in my cell and pleaded that the Dy. Superintendent was all praise for me and I should pay more attention to his case. He told me that the D.I.G. Prisons had heavily punished him for a very small act of negligence. He had been demoted from Dy. Superintendent to Asst. Superintendent and that his piles too had aggravated since then. I took the clue and prescribed IGNATIA. This remedy acts wonderfully in ailments which follow grief, disappointment, worry, despair, mental shock or mortification. I need not say that IGNATIA cured the patient not only physically but mentally also.

Many children become irritable, they want to be carried in the lap and are obstinate, easily angered. A few globules of CHAMOMILLA 6, 12 wonderfully calm such children. This remedy is often called the opium of Homoeopathy, ACID PHOS works very well in the ailments of disappointed lovers. AURUM (gold subsides thoughts of suicide and disgust for life.

Once a Member of Parliament consulted me. He said that for the last 3-4 weeks he had been feeling afraid of making any speech in Parliament, though all along he had been a good speaker. This is called stage-fright. A dose of GELSEMIUM 200 totally removed this fright in him.

One Executive Engineer developed a strange sense of anguish and despondency which lasted only for about 2 hours in the morning. He felt he will not be able to work in the office, he will be unable to deal with the files. There was great tension in the morning but when he went to the office he was quite normal and the same tension returned the next morning. A dose of ARSENICUM ALBUM 1,000 relieved his tension in three days only.

6

DOSE AND SELECTING POTENCY

Homoeopathic medicines are available in four forms:

- Mother Tinctures
- Pillules
- Globules and
- Triturations (Powder)

Mother Tinctures are extracts of original remedies prepared mostly in alcohol. Pillules are made of cane sugar which are then absorbed with a few drops of liquid medicine. These are kept in small bottles and are quite easy to handle. Globules are smaller than pillules, and Triturations are in the form of powder or tablets made from powder which contains the medicine triturated with sugar of milk.

Pillules and globules may be taken dry on tongue or sucked but should not be swallowed. These could also be dissolved in pure water and taken. Triturations should be taken dry on the tongue. One should clean his mouth before taking a medicine.

Ordinarily the dose of a liquid medicine is one drop in an ounce of pure water for an adult, for children 1/2 drop and for babies 1/4 drop. If the medicine is in tritruations, i.e., powder form, 3-4 grains for adults, 2 for children and 1 grain for babies is quite sufficient.

Pills or globules can be prepared of all the liquid medicines. Take a small phial, fill two thirds of it with globules or pills and saturate these pills with a few drops of the liquid medicine. Shake well. These globules may be given 1 or 2 to babies, 2 to 3 to children and 4 to 5 to adults.

REPETITION OF DOSES: The dose is repeated according to the severity of the disease. For example, in cholera we can repeat the medicine hourly, half-hourly and even quarter-hourly. In ordinary diseases, doses may be repeated 4 to 6 hours. In chronic ailments, medicines are given once a week or even once a month or so.

SELECTION OF POTENCY: This is a very ticklish question. There are no prescribed rules for selection of potencies, but ordinarily low potencies such as 3X, 3, 6, 6X or 30 are used in acute diseases, but in chronic diseases high potencies such as 200, 500, 1,000 are used at long intervals. The highest potencies such as 10M, 50M, CM are given in very chronic diseases at intervals of several weeks or even months.

IS AN ANTIDOTE NEEDED? When a patient begins Homoeopathic treatment, it is not always necessary to give him some medicine to antidote the effects of the previous medicines. Generally NUX VOM. 30 to 200 one dose is said to antidote all other medicinal effects. But only time neutralises the effects of drugs. If the case is not acute and urgent a dose of NUX may be given to start with.

7

TRY HOMOEOPATHY TO AVOID SURGERY

We have explained in brief the principles of Homoeopathic science, but we find that there are many misunderstandings in the minds of even well educated persons. We should therefore want to remove these as far as possible.

It is often said that there is no surgery in Homoeopathy and without it, it cannot be called a complete science. This is a great misunderstanding. Homoeopathy is a therapeutic science or the art of healing the diseases of human beings by using medicinal substances. Surgery is a technique, a method of removing certain impediments in the way of curing a disease, such as removing a thorn from one's foot, or setting up a dislocated bone. If a foreign particle has entered one's eye, we would have to remove the foreign body by washing the eye by using an eyeglass, or if we turn over the lid and clear the eye with a wet linen, the foreign body will be removed. There cannot be two opinions about it. All sciences whether it is Allopathy, Homoeopathy, or Ayurveda, will take the same step. Therefore, where this kind of manipulation or surgery is needed, Homoeopathy will agree to it.

But there is a difference of opinion regarding where surgery would be essential and where it could be avoided. *We are of the opinion that in 50 per cent of the cases where surgery is practised it can safely be avoided.* As soon as a case of tonsilitis or appendicitis is detected, Allopathy would at once advise surgery, but I can say from my own experience that many cases of appendix and tonsils have been completely cured by oral medicines, though there have been such cases of appendix and tonsils or fistula in which I myself have advised operation. Cases of gangrene declared incurable and advised amputation of the affected limb, yielded to Homoeopathic treatment and the patients are hale and hearty. Therefore no system of medicine can be called incomplete if it does not have surgery. It fact, surgery is common to all medical systems.

Often patients ask Homoeopaths: "Doctor, can Homoeopathy treat a case of Asthma?" "Are there remedies for liver troubles in Homoeopathy?" "Can enlarged prostates be cured by medicines without operation?" There is only one answer to all such questions that Homoeopathy can successfully treat and cure all such cases. It will, therefore, be wiser to give it a trial.

II

CURES

We now give symptoms of diseases and their remedies with distinctive symptoms or characteristics of each. Laymen and housewives can select and cure ordinary ailments with the help of this guide. In serious cases, a Homoeopath of your city or town should be consulted.

It should again be underlined that Homoeopathy does not treat diseases as they are classified in other systems of medicine, but the symptoms that occur in various diseases. In a single disease there may be a large variety of cases with altogether different symptoms. Therefore the reader is advised to check these as carefully as he possibly can with the symptoms of various medicines indicated in that disease before finally selecting the medicine.

For this reason, medicines are indicated in bolder type and acquire a prominent place in this books. This should not confuse the reader because it is from these various medicines that he has to select his own. Moreover, nearly all the medicines are used in many diseases which should again not confuse the reader. In Homoeopathy one medicine is used in many diseases.

8

FEVERS

The normal temperature of the human body is 98.4 °F or 37 °C. When the thermometer after putting it for a minute or so in the mouth below the tongue shows a rise in temperature it is termed fever. The body becomes hot and the pulse rate increase in proportion of 10 to 1 degree rise in temperature. Respiration increases generally by 2 to 1 degree of temperature. Rise of temperature above 105 degrees and fall below 96 are both dangerous.

In fact, fever in itself is not a disease but it occurs when there is a disease. When some derangement occurs in our body, Nature or our Vital Force tries to set right the derangement, and fever is a symptom of that effort of Nature. Hence fevers should not be got rid of by drastic medicines, but effort should be made to remove the cause of the fever. It often occurs when there is an inflammation or swelling in any part of the body. Fever also occurs when toxins or some foreign poisonous matter gets into the blood stream. Severe cold, heat of the sun, great weariness, etc. also result in fever. For such fevers the following medicines should be given according to the cause and symptoms.

- ACONITE 3x or 30: This medicine if given in the beginning

will subside many fevers caused by the heat of the sun, getting wet in the rain, getting chilled from dry cold wind, etc. The patient of Aconite is restless, he fears he will die, his skin is dry and hot, he feels thirsty and anguished, and gets worse in the night. In the beginning give him a drop in water or 3-4 globules dry on the tongue, every 2 or 3 hours. Stop it if the fever falls and the patient starts perspiring.

- BELLADONNA 3X or 30: For high fever, severe headache, face red and flushed, throbbing blood vessels, red eyes, fat flabby persons.
- DULCAMARA: For fever in rainy season on account of the damp atmosphere or getting wet in rain.
- PULSATILLA: For fever due to overeating or too much bathing. No thirst. Patient tearful.
- CAMPHOR: When the fever is caused by catching cold, one or two drops of mother tincture (Q) with a little sugar of milk will avert it. Bruised pain all over the body and chill are its particular symptoms. If one has to go out in severe winter a dose or two of CAMPHOR Q will protect him from catching cold.
- GELSEMIUM: The patient lies dull, with closed eyes, little thirst, pain in body specially in back, partial unconsciousness.
- FERRUM PHOS 6X TRIT.: Slight fever, the patient is neither restless like ACONITE nor dull like GBLS. 5 tablets or 5 grains of powder with hot water will avert many fevers if given early every 2 to 3 hours.
- BRYONIA: Pain in head and limbs, getting worse even on slight movement. Breathing difficult, cough, great thirst for large quantities of water at long intervals. Taste bitter, constipation, tongue dirty or yellowish.
- RHUS TOX.: Extreme restlessness, patient turns sides frequently. fever due to getting wet in rain or chilling in wet cold wind. Pain all over the body, much pain in back, pain in joints, tongue dirty, but tip is red.

- ARSENIC ALB: Thirst for small quantities but frequently. Worse after midnight, restlessness, anguish, feeling of burning, diarrhoea, extreme prostration. It is often needed in later stages.

MALARIA

This is an intermittent fever the symptoms of which are common knowledge. Generally fever begins with chill, often severe chill, which may last for minutes or even a few hours. After the chill, fever rises and sometimes it is as high as 104° or 105°; after a few hours the patient perspires and fever comes down to normal. This paroxysm is repeated the same time next day or after two or three days. When the fever attacks daily, it is called Quotidian, and when it recurs after 48 hours it is called Tertian and when after 72 hours it is Quartan. Sometimes both chill and perspiration or one of these are absent. This fever is caused by a particular mosquito which injects material parasites into the blood.

Cinchona or Quinine kills these parasites and thus in Allopathy it is the remedy of all sorts of material fevers. Many different preparations of Quinine (Camoquine, Chloroquine, Plasmoquine) are available in the market and are extensively used in malaria. 3 or 4 tablets daily often check the malarial paroxysms, but often fever reappears after some time. For a complete and radical cure of malaria Homoeopathic medicines are the best, but you will have to select the medicine exactly according to the symptoms of the patient such as the time of chill and fever; symptoms during fever — thirst, restlessness, pains, etc., and other general and particular symptoms of the patient. Here are the symptoms of some of the important medicines.

- IPECAC: When gastric symptoms predominate, such as nausea, heaviness of stomach, salivation, vomiting, bitter taste, and the time of fever is generally between 9 to 11 p.m.; chill for a few minutes but fever last longer, chill is aggravated in a warm room or hot drink produces oppression in the chest. It is claimed that if the symptoms are not clear, two or three doses of IPECAC will either cure the patient or the symptoms will become more prominent which will help selection of the right remedy. It is also useful when fever persists even after QUININE or ARSENIC is taken. It also cures the effects of the abuse of QUININE.

- ARSENICUM ALBUM: The time of fever is generally after 12 a.m. or 12 p.m. All the three stages are not marked; chill and heat are mixed or alternated. In chronic cases when liver and spleen are affected. The patient drinks a little but too often. Anguish, anxiety, a burning feeling but the patient wants to cover himself. Great restlessness, great prostration. The patient is weak and emaciated even during apyrexia. The Tertian and Quartan fevers yield to this remedy readily as well as fevers which occur twice every day. In the beginning use 3x potency every 4 hours or so, but in chronic cases give 200 or 1000 and during apyrexia at least 2 doses.
- CHINA or CINCHONA: Thirst before and during chill; chill begins from feet and spreads all over the body. Thirst but drinking chills the patient. Time of chill is about 5 a.m. or 5 p.m.; liver and spleen are enlarged. Sweats in the night, weekly fever with nausea and vomiting.
- NATRUM MURIATICUM: This is a sure remedy when the symptoms are the following. Time of chill is between 9 a.m. to 11 a.m., fever continues from 4 to 5 hours and is down by 4 to 5 p.m. Face of the patient is smooth or oily. There is often noted a crack in the middle of the lower lip. Patient is sad, morose and anxious, often tearful. Consolation aggravates, nausea, vomiting and other usual symptoms. Liver and spleen enlarged, taste bitter. Quotidian, Tertian or Quartan all fevers come under this remedy. It should be given in 6x or 30 during

fever and 200 or 1000 during apyrexia or when the fever is lowest.

- NUX VOMICA: Time of chill 8 a.m. to 11 a.m. Chilly even during fever, wants to be covered during fever, gastric symptoms predominate, nausea, vomiting, bitter taste, aggravation from open air. During chill lips and nails become blue; liver and spleen are affected.
- SULPHUR: Time of chill morning or 4 p.m., late evening, chill even during fever. Craves open air. Likes neither cold nor heat. Fevers that begin at 10p.m. are readily cured by 2 or 3 doses of SULPHUR Q one drop each dose.
- CHININUM ARS: Fever rises in the afternoon. Extreme debility, wants to sit by fire, likes hot drink. Give 3x every 2 hours during apyrexia.
- FERRUM PHOS: Time of chill is about 1 p.m. Fever lasts for 3-4 hours. Cold sweats in the night. Give 200x or 1000 during apyrexia every 3 hours.
- LACHESIS: Time of fever is between 2 p.m. to 4 p.m., chill is legs and back. Hot sweating even during fever, aggravation after rising from sleep. Patient is talkative, liver and spleen are effected, bleeding from nose.
- THUJA: Time 3 a.m. or 3 p.m. Sweats on uncovered portion of the body only, chill in thighs.
- SYPHILINUM: Time 10-11 p.m., and is down by 5 or 6 a.m. 200 or 1000 potency be given twice in the day.
- PYROGEN: Time 7 p.m. Offensive sweat, stools and breath. During fever patient is talkative. Pulse is proportionately rapid. Sweats without relief in fever, which rises even after sweating.
- CEDRON: Fever exactly at the same time every day, so much so that you can adjust your watch. Often the time of fever is midday. Give 2 drops of every 2 hours starting about 8 or 6 hours before the time of fever.
- NATRUM SULPH: Time 5 a.m. or 5 p.m. Bitter taste, worse from water or watery fruits such as melons. Liver enlarged, vomiting.

- FERRUM METALICUM: Time 4 a.m. Patient is anaemic, pale face, vomits whatever he eats; epistaxis, liver effected, pain all over the body during fever.
- PULSATILLA: Time of chill morning, afternoon or evening. Complete absence of thirst, the patient likes cold air. Weeps easily, feels chilly but is worsened by heat. Sometimes the fever rises twice every day. Sometimes feels heat and sweats in half of the body only.
- LYCOPODIUM: Time of chill is 4 or 5 p.m. and often the fever comes down by 8-9 p.m. Often sweats immediately after chill. Does not want to be covered. Gases in the abdomen. Urine is dark and scanty. 200 or 1000 potency repeated 2-3 times during the day will avert fever.
- CALCAREA CARB: Time of chill between 2 and 3 p.m. Fever rises with chill. Knees and feet feel cold and wet; sweat mostly on head, neck and chest.
- APIS MEL: Time of chill 3 p.m. No thirst, does not want to be covered, worse from heat. Urine dark and scanty. Urticaria, thirst during chill and craves cold water. Not much sweating.
- CHELIDONIUM: Time of chill between 4 a.m. and 8 a.m. or 4 p.m. Chill and sweating not much, fever high, vomits, better with hot drinks, worse with cold water. Headache on right half, jaundice. Pain in back below the right scapula.
- PODOPHYLLUM: Time of chill between 6 to 8 a.m. Talks much during fever, pain in joints and back during chill. Sweats much and sleeps during sweats, when fever is down.
- VERATRUM ALBUM: Time is 6 to 8 a.m. Cold, sweats on forehead and limbs. Cramps in limbs. Body cold.
- EUPATORIUM PERFOLIATUM: Severe pain in bones all over. No thirst during chill but much before and after. Nausea and vomiting, scanty sweating.
- CACTUS: Time 11 a.m. or 11 p.m. Chill even during fever. Feels palpitation and dyspnoea.

- ALSTONIA: Time 9 and 11 a.m. Liver and spleen effected, diarrhoea or dysentery.
- BAPTISIA: Time 11 a.m. to 12. Offensive stools, pain in the body, diarrhoea.
- MALARIA OFFICINALIS: Time after midday. Old cases when fever recurs again and again, sweats scanty. During malarial season use 30 or 200 potency twice a week as preventive.

Chill Time and the Medicine

Since Chill Time is very important in this fever, select the medicine as follows:

1 p.m. - FERRUM PHOS.
2 p.m. - CALC CARB, LACHESIS
3 p.m. - APIS, CHIN. S.
3-4 p.m. - LYCO., THUJA
4-8 p.m. - LYCO.
5 p.m. - CHINA
Forenoon - N.V., CHINA
Seventh day - CHINA
Midday - GELS.
Midnight - ARS., NUX V.
1-2 a.m. - ARS.
3 a.m. - THUJA
4 a.m. - FEBRRUM MET.
5 a.m. - CHINA
6-7 a.m. - PODOPHYLLUM
7-9 a.m. - EUP. PERF.
9-11 a.m. - NAT M.
11 a.m.- 11 p.m. - CACTUS
Periodic - ARNICA, CEDRON, CHIN. S., IPECAC.
Every Spring - LACHESIS

TYPHOID FEVER

Typhoid fever is called enteric fever, fever of the intestines. There is no remission in this fever. In typhoid the pulse rate does not increase to the extent it should normally increase with temperature, i.e., about 10-12 times with 1 degree rise of temperature. In the morning the temperature falls down daily but increases about 2 degrees in the afternoon and evening. The tongue is invariably coated thick. Generally 21 days is the period of this fever but sometimes it comes down in 14 days and sometimes takes about 40 to 42 days. Some remittent fevers come down in seven days only. Constipation during the fever is a good sign; diarrhoea may create complications. Nowadays in Allopathy the use of antibiotic drugs brings down the temperature in 4 or 5 days but sometimes other complications arise. Properly selected Homoeopathic medicines too often cut short the attack and prevent complications. Complete rest, a liquid diet and proper nursing is essential in this.

- BRYONIA: This in the head remedy of this fever. Often small white or red pimple like eruptions are seen on the neck, chest and abdomen in the second week of this fever. The temperature falls when the eruptions come down the chest. BRYONIA helps in bringing out these eruptions. Constipation, hard stools, thirst at long intervals but for large quantities of water are characteristic symptoms in BRYONIA. The patient is not restless and wants to lie down silently; motion aggravates his malady. Two or three doses of 30 potency daily should be given.
- RHUS TOX.: Symptoms opposed to BRYONIA. The patient is restless and often changes position in bed. Tongue is coated but the tip is red.
- BAPTISIA: Mother tincture of this remedy, a drop for a dose, 3 or 4 times daily is very effective in this disease. It is the chief remedy of typhoid. It controls even

diarrhoea. Keeps the intestines safe and averts all complications. It can be given in alteration with other indicated remedies.

- ARSENIC ALB.: From the very beginning the patient is extremely restless and prostrated. Thirst for small quantities of water at very short intervals. Anguish.
- HELLEBORUS and HYOSCYAMUS: These medicines are useful when there is a brain complication. The patient is unconscious or is delirious. GELSEMIUM, OPIUM, ARSENIC are also indicated in this disease. Boiled water should be given and milk also should be diluted with water. Even after the fever is down, solid food should be avoided for a week or two.

MEASLES

This is a very contagious disease. It generally occurs during spring. If a child in a family is attacked by measles, nearly all children are attacked sooner or later. The exact nature of the poison is not known but after the poison gets into the blood in a week or two, the disease begins with cold, coryza, fever and cough. After 3 or 4 days a red rash appears on the face and all over the body. Fever sometimes rises up to 103°-104°. After the appearance of rash the fever subsides in a day or two. Cough often persists even after the temperature comes down to normal. Sometimes the cold sets in the lungs and bronchitis or pneumonia may occur. High fever, diarrhoea or delirium are not good symptoms.

- ACONITE: ACONITE 3x should be given as soon as cold, watering from the nose and eyes or fever is detected. Thirst, restlessness, chilliness are felt by the patient.
- BELLADONNA 3x or 30: Face red, fever high, severe headache, pain in throat, startles during sleep, eyes red, thirst.
- PULSATILLA 6, 30: Thirstless, cough in the evening or

night, diarrhoea, loose motions, thick, yellowish discharge from nose.

- BRYONIA 3x or 30: Thirst for large quantities at long intervals, dry cough. If the rash is suppressed BRYONIA will bring it out.
- GELSIMIUM: Suppression of rash, high fever.
- FERRUM PHOS. 6x TRIT.: Could be given in all stages of the disease. 3-4 grains with hot water.
- ANTIM TART. 3x TRIT. or 6: When lungs are involved in bronchitis or pneumonia.
- MURBILINUM 30: Can be used in all stages. As measles is mostly a children's disease, two globules of this remedy will act as prophylactic and protect children from its attack when there is the epidemic, during spring in particular. A dose of PULSATILLA 30 twice a week will also act as prophylactic.

SMALL POX

This is also a very contagious disease and like measles generally attacks children. Its incubation period (the time between the entering of poison in the body and appearance of fever, etc.) is 10-12 days. The fever often goes as high as 105° and 108°F. 5-6 days after fever there are red eruptions all over the body. Within 4-5 days pus is formed and all eruptions contain pus. These eruptions often cover not only the whole body but even the tongue, inner mouth and throat, eyes, nose, etc. If the eruptions are close to each other the disease is considered to be serious. Ordinarily after 10-12 days these eruptions fade, pus is dried up and fever comes down. Those children who are vaccinated do not get this disease or even if it attacks, the attack is mild.

Any of the three Homoeopathic medicines, VARIOLINUM 30, VICCININUM 30, MALANDRINUM 30, can be given twice a week, and if there is some fever, it should be regarded as having served the purpose of vaccination.

- VARIOLINUM 30: Should be given twice a week to children or adults. It will protect them from the attack of small pox during the epidemic. Among Hindus small pox is regarded as Goddess Shitala who rides on an ass. Science says that asses are immune to small pox and the milk of she-ass protects people from small pox.

In the beginning BELLADONNA, BAPTISIA should be given. If lungs are involved VERATRUM VIRIDE is suggested. These medicines should be used according to their symptoms. After the eruptions come out, THUJA, RHUS TOX. should be given. If lungs are attacked ANTIM. TART. is the best remedy.

- SARRACENIA: Can be given in all stages, its use averts the disease and face damage is prevented. ANTIM. TART. or MERC. SOL. is given after pus is formed. Sometimes the eruptions are completely or partially suppressed, but this is not a good symptom; SULPHUR, CAMPHOR or THUJA should be studied in such cases. To save face damage the patient should be protected from sunlight or even electric light, and red curtains and red bulbs should be used. The bedding and clothes of the patient should either be burnt or disinfected in boiling water for some days. When the eruptions dry up, there is great itching, and olive oil or carbolic oil should be applied to these. Sometimes some skin diseases appear after vaccination; THUJA and KALI MUR. are the best antidotes of this poison. Use of these will protect one from the bad effects of vaccination. THUJA 200 once a week will do. KALI MUR. 6X can be given one dose daily for some days.

9

DISEASES OF THE DIGESTIVE ORGANS

COLIC (PAIN IN ABDOMEN)

Pain in abdomen is very common; it occurs due to various causes, such as indigestion, gases, acidity, flatulence, constipation, worms, etc. The root of all these is poor digestion and our inability to assimilate the food taken.

Therefore, as soon as pain in abdomen is felt, all food should be stopped and hot water should be taken frequently. No food should be taken during the pain. Sometimes pain occurs on account of cold. Hot fomentation of the abdomen is advisable.

- MAGNESIA PHOS 3X: Powder or tablets should be given dissolved in half a cup of hot water. If the pain is severe, the medicine may be repeated every half hour or 15 minutes. In a majority of cases 2-3 doses will relieve all sorts of pain.
- COLOCYNTHIS: When there is pain in and around the navel and the patient bends double due to pain. It gets better when pressed with hand. 6, 30 should be repeated hourly. Also when it is worse after anger.

- NUX VOM.: When the pain is accompanied by constipation.
- DIOSCOREA: When the pain starting from the centre of the abdomen shifts to different parts, even fingers and toes. When there is rumbling with passing of much flatus, worse on bending forward, better on walking or bending backward.
- CHAMOMILLA: When the pain is gripping around the navel, there is diarrhoea, and the pain is worse in the night and with heat.
- LYCO.: When there is rumbling, the patient passes flatus, it gets worse between 4-8 p.m., there is flatulence.
- PULSATILLA: When there is pain due to taking of rich food, the patient is thirstless, has a weeping mood, dry tongue but no thirst, or pain during menses.
- IRIS V.: When there is gripping, vomiting of bile, and flatulence.
- VERATRUM ALBUM: When there is pain after the evening meal and rumbling.

DYSPEPSIA OR INDIGESTION

Loss of appetite, flatulence, non-digestion of food, at times constipation and at times diarrhoea, salivation, a dull pain in the abdomen, nausea, sour eructations, frequent urine, pain in hands and legs, and various other symptoms are found in this disease. The main cause is irregularity in life, unwholesome food and lack of exercise.

Fatty rich food should be stopped at once, only fruit diet for a week or so will restore health. One or two meals should be missed every week. A morning walk in open air for 2-3 miles is necessary. Food should be regulated and intervals increased.

- PULSATILLA: When there is a salty taste and no thirst, or it is due to taking ice-cream or fatty rich food.

- NATRUM MUR.: When there is anaemia and a craving for salt. When it gets worse on taking potatoes or bread, or due to overindulgence, when it gets worse at about 11 a.m. to 5 p.m. Nausea, chilliness and burning in the stomach.
- SULPHUR: When there is constipation, piles, the patient is hungry in the night. For chronic cases.
- ARSENIC: When there is great thirst or it occurs due to ice-cream.
- LYCO.: When it is due to flatulence or overindulgence, gets worse about 4 to 8 p.m.
- ABILES NIGRA: When there is pain immediately after taking food. Suits old persons.
- CARBO VEG.: When there are eructations, pain in chest, hands and feet are cold.
- CALCAREA CARB.: When there are sour eructations. For chronic cases. Suits fat and flabby patients.
- HEPAR: When there is craving for sour food.
- NUX MOSCH: When the patient has pain after meals, or it is due to suppression of skin diseases.
- ANACARDIUM: When the malady is relieved by taking food but symptoms reappear after a few hours.
- NATRUM PHOS.: When there is acidity or it is due to worms.
- CHINA: When it is due to over drinking or frequent attacks of malaria.
- IODIUM: When it is with increased appetite.
- ZINGIBER: When it is due to contaminated water or watery fruits such as melons, etc.
- ANTIM CRUD.: When the patient has thick white-coated tongue, heaviness in the abdomen, nausea, vomits bile mucus.
- KALI BICHROM: When it is due to over drinking of beer, the patient has a craving for acidic things, aversion to water, it gets worse after taking food.

- GENTIANA: When there is a loss of appetite. Take doses of 2 drops half an hour before meals.

Acidity is generally the main cause of dyspepsia. Therefore acidic things should be avoided, soda water is useful.

CONSTIPATION

It is a common complaint. Purgatives should not be taken. Though they relieve for the time being, they do not cure the tendency. Moreover, when liquid stools are passed with their use, many vitamins are lost and the patient becomes weak.

Constipation can arise from organic causes, such as narrowing of the bowel and obstruction from growths, but the vast majority of constipation cases stem from easily modified causes, such as:

- A diet lacking in fiber or fluids.
- Lack of exercise.
- Negative emotional state.
- Ignoring the signal to move the bowels.

You can prevent constipation by changing above habits. However, according to the nature of constipation the following medicines may be used:

- NUX VOM.: When the patient has to go twice or thrice in the morning to toilet as the stool is not cleared, one dose of 30 may be taken before going to bed for a few days.
- BRYONIA: When there is no urge for stools; stools are dry and difficult, and there is much thirst.
- ALUMINA: When there is dryness in intestines, no urge for days until there is a great accumulation. Small balls like stools, evacuation difficult, one has to exert.
- OPIUM: No stools for days but the patient does not feel

any uneasiness. It would seem that the intestines have stopped functioning. Round, hard, black balls.

- PLUMBUM: Chief remedy for chronic constipation. There is an urge but stools pass with difficulty. Hard, lumpy, black stools.
- NATRUM MUR., GRAPHITES, MAGNESIA MUR. and CAUSTICUM should also be considered.

DIARRHOEA

Continuous watery stools with or without pain is called diarrhoea.

- NUX VOM.: When it occurs after heavy meals, there are frequent stools, yet the patient feels that the motion is not clear.
- SPIRIT CAMPHOR Q: When it occurs during hot summer days; hands and feet are cold and the patient is chilly. 2-3 drops in sugar once or twice will give relief.
- PULSATILLA: When it is due to rich fatty food and there is rumbling. No two stools are alike in colour and it gets worse on consuming fruits.
- CHINA: When there are watery motions without pain. Extreme prostration. Much thirst, perspiration all over. When it occurs after taking fruits.
- ALOE: When it is due to beer, there are forcibly shot out watery stools, stool passes unnoticed. When the urging is imperative.
- ARSENIC: When there is unquenchable thirst, the patient feels restless, painful, burning.
- VERATRUM ALB.: When there are cramps in the abdomen, white watery stools which pass unnoticed, body gets cold, there is cold sweat and much thirst.
- CROTON: When there are yellowish watery stools forcibly shot out, nausea, gets worse on taking food or drink and better on taking hot water.

- CHAMOMILLA: When there are greenish, watery, hot, offensive stools, and cramp in abdomen. For diarrhoea of teething children, child very irritable.
- ACONITE: When it is due to dry cold, anger, fear or suppression of perspiration.
- ANTIM CRUD.: When there is irritability, white-coated tongue, diarrhoea alternates with constipation.
- CALCAREA CARB.: When there are whitish stools with sour smell; suits fair, fat, flabby patients.
- CALCAREA PHOS.: When it occurs during dentition and gets worse in the morning.
- PODOPHYLLUM: When there are profuse offensive stools. For children during dentition, child's cheek becomes red and hot when washed.
- RHEUM: For sour stools during dentition sour smell from the body of the child. Colour of stool becomes greenish after a few minutes.
- SULPHUR: In chronic cases which get worse in the mornings. Urging imperative, drives the patient out of bed.

CHRONIC DIARRHOEA

Sometimes ordinary diarrhoea takes a chronic turn and lasts for months and years. There is little pain but the patient is unable to digest anything. He passes loose watery stools many times. In addition to the medicines already given under diarrhoea the following should be studied and tried.

- CHAPARRO AMARGOSO Q. When there is tenderness over liver, stools with little pain but much mucus. Acts as tonic. Mother tincture or 3 potency be used for sometime.
- VACCINIUM MYRTILLUS Q: Keeps intestines aseptic and prevents reabsorption and reinfection.
- CALCAREA CARB, CALCAREA PHOS. are also useful.

DYSENTERY

Infection of the intestines resulting in severe diarrhoea with the presence of blood and mucus in the faeces.

- MERC SOL. and MERC CORR.: These are the chief remedies. The patient feels he has not evacuated — this never got done feeling is the chief symptom. There is salivation in the mouth. When there is more of blood, prescribe MERC CORR., and when there is more of mucus, give MERC SOL.
- ACONITE: When it is due to dry cold wind, there is fever, fear of death and restlessness.
- NUX VOM.: When pain subsides after passing of stools but reappears after some time. In MERC SOL. the pain and urging remains constant and in NUX it disappears for some time.
- TROMBIDIUM: When there is much pain before and after stools and it gets worse by taking food or drink.
- SULPHUR: In chronic cases, when there is a red line of blood in stools.
- RHUS TOX.: When there is great restlessness, or it occurs in rainy season.

CHOLERA

This is an acute infectious disease characterised by violent vomiting, purging, cramps and collapse. The exciting cause is generally considered to be the Comma Bacillus, which was discovered by Koch who came to India in 1883, deputed by the German government. In cholera the patient gets thirsty but urine is suppressed inspite of the great intake of water.

- CAMPHOR Q (SPIRIT CAMPHOR): It has proved very efficacious in the treatment of cholera. Fifty per cent cases of cholera are nipped in the bud by giving 2-3 drops of it in sugar every hour or half hour according to the seriousness of symptoms. Cold hands and feet, cold sweats and coldness all over are its chief symptoms.

- ARSENIC: When there is unquenchable thirst, very frequent, but the patient takes little and wants it again after a few minutes. Vomiting, cold sweat, burning, extreme restlessness and prostration, fear of death are also there. Aggravation after midnight.
- IPECAC: When there is constant nausea and vomiting, the tongue is red.
- VERATRUM ALBUM: When there is rapid pulse, white motions, unquenchable thirst, cramps, spasms, cold sweats, specially on forehead. Body cold and bluish, tongue cold.
- CUPRUM MET.: When there are brown, dark, greenish stools, lips cold and blue, eyes sunken, dark circles around eyes, cramps, colic, and urine is suppressed.
- CARBO VEG.: When the patient feels very hot, wants to be fanned though the body is cold.
- AETHUSA: When there is prostration and sleep after vomiting, specially in children.
- ANTIM TART.: When there is cold sweat, irritability, the child does not like to be touched or even looked at.
- SECALE: When the fingers are bent backwards on account of cramps, the body is cold but does not like to be covered. The patient feels great burning, wants to be fanned.
- PULSATILLA: When it occurs after taking rich, heavy fatty food or ice cream or fruits. The patient is thirstless, weeps easily, the colour of motions changes every time.
- PHOSPHORUS: When there are gushing stools, anus seems to remain open and stool passes constantly, water is vomited as soon as it is taken.
- CANTHARIS: When urine is not passing though it collects in the bladder.
- TEREBINTHINA: When urine is totally suppressed and the bladder is empty.

- RHUS TOX.: In extreme restlessness, the patient turns side to side.
- IRIS: When there are motions with a sour smell.

In cholera often dehydration takes place. Saline water is then given intravenously which is very useful. Salt is given dissolved in drinking water.

VOMITING

- IPECAC: When there is constant nausea, food is vomited, the tongue is red.
- ANTIM CRUD.: When the tongue is thick, white coated.
- ROBINIA: When there is sour vomiting.
- ARSENIC: When there is burning in the stomach, debility, thirst, vomiting due to an ulcer in the stomach, restlessness.
- AETHUSA: When there is vomiting of curdled milk in children, and they sleep after the vomit.
- KREOSOTE: When it occurs during pregnancy or hysteria.
- APOMORPHIA: For vomiting of pregnant women or addicts of alcohol or opium.
- ARNICA: When it occurs due to injury to head.
- COCCULUS: For vomiting in ship, boat, bus, train or car.
- MILLEFOLIUM: When there is vomiting of red blood.
- HAMAMELIS: When there is vomiting of dark blood.
- PHOSPHORUS: When cold water is vomited as soon as it becomes warm in stomach.
- NUX VOM.: When there is bilious or acid vomiting.

ACIDITY

It is a symptom of indigestion. There is abnormal acid in stomach, which results in sour eructations, burning, and pain in abdomen. Acid fruits and sour things should be avoided soda-bicarb or soda water should be taken.

- CALCAREA CARB.: Chief remedy, specially suited to fat, flabby persons.
- SULPHURIC ACID 6, 30: When there is hiccough, sour smell from the body, burning and sour eructations.
- ROBINIA: When there is sour sweat, greenish vomit, burning, sour eructations.
- NATRUM PHOS. 6X: Very effective. Take powder or tablets dry on tongue 2-3 times a day.
- ARGENTUM NIT.: When the appetite is increased, there is craving for sweet things, eructations.
- KALI CARB.: Suitable for old persons.
- CARBO VEG.: When there are gases in abdomen, eructations.
- LYCO.: When there is dark urine, flatulence.
- SULPHUR: In chronic cases.

GASTRIC ULCER

Due to acidity the mucus membrane of stomach is often ulcerated. There is pain and burning. The pain is often relieved by taking some food but after some time it recurs.

- HYDRASTIS 6 or 30: The head remedy. Medicines suggested under acidity should be tried.
- NATRUM PHOS, SULPHURIC ACID, ANACARDIUM, KALI BICH. are also indicated.

HICCOUGH

In serious diseases hiccough is often indicative of collapse. If the hiccough is hysteric or dyspeptic, patient is not serious, it is easily controlled.

- GINSENG Q: Best remedy. 2 drops, 3-4 times, with a little water.
- NUX VOM.: When it is due to indigestion.
- COCCULUS: When hunger is gone, there is disgust for food, gets worse riding a car, bus, boat, etc.
- CUPRUM: When it is due to spasm, with nausea.
- IGNATIA: When it is due to smoking.
- NATRUM MUR.: Use it for malarial patients.
- LYCO.: When the tongue comes out and then contracts and goes in.
- CICUTA: When there is a loud sound.

GALL COLIC

The liver secretes bile which is stored in the gall-bladder. Sometimes stone is formed in the bladder and when it moves and passes in blood vessels, there is severe pain.

- CALCAREA CARB.: 30 or 200 should be given every 15-20 minutes during the attack.
- BERBERIS V. Q: 5 drops with an ounce of warm water be repeated hourly or half hourly.
- MAGNESIA PHOS. 3X: 5 grains or 5 tablets with hot water every half hour.
- CHELIDONIUM Q AND HYDRASTIS Q: These will also relieve pain when given in doses of 5 drops with hot water.
- CHOLESTERINUM 3: Should be given to bring out the stone.
- BERBERIS Q: Twice daily will bring out the stone.
- CHINA Q or 6: Will bring out the stone when used for some days twice daily.
- CARDUUS M. Q: These medicines are also useful.

APPENDICITIS

On the right side, in our abdomen, at the junction of the small intestines with large intestines, there is a fingerlike organ called appendix. It becomes inflamed and painful and the pain recurs again and again after days or weeks. In acute cases there is fever, severe pain, restlessness, nausea, vomiting, etc. Sometimes suppuration occurs and pus is formed in the appendix. In such serious cases the organ is removed by operation. Homoeopathic medicines if taken, can subside the acute attack and cure the appendix.

- ACONITE: To be given in the beginning when there is high fever.
- BELLADONNA: Chief remedy of the disease. To be given when there is severe pain which gets worse on lying, red face, high fever.
- BRYONIA: When there is sticking pain, constipation, thirst, fever, etc. and the patient gets relief by lying on the right side.
- LACHESIS: When the patient cannot bear to be touched at the painful spot.
- APIS: When there is severe pain, no thirst.
- IRISTENAX 30: Will prevent recurrence when given a dose daily for some time.
- MERC. SOL.: When pus is likely to be formed, pain gets worse by lying on the right side.
- HEPAR, COLOCYNTH and SULPHUR are also used.

PILES

In this disease the blood vessels of the anus swell and haemorrhoids are formed which are painful and also bleed. When bleeding occurs, it is called bleeding piles and when there is pain but no blood, it is called blind piles

- NUX and SULPHUR: Both these medicines have proved very efficacious in this disease. A dose of NUX 30 at bed time and one of SULPHUR 30 in the morning will cure 60 per cent cases of both the types.

- COLLINSONIA 3X: Specially suitable for pregnant women.
- AESCULUS: When there is pain in rectum and back, the patient feels as if a splinter is fixed in the rectum. When there are haemorrhoids outside anus.
- HAMAMELIS Q 6, 30: When there is bleeding of dark blood. It can be used externally as ointment mixed with vaseline.
- RATANHIA Q or 6: When there is severe pain lasting for hours after passing stools, the patient feels as if pieces of broken glass were in the rectum. Fissures. The patient is better by cold applications.
- GRAPHITES: When there is constipation, fissures, long lasting pain after stools as if someone was cutting with a knife.
- ALOE: When there are loose motions, bleeding and cutting pain.
- PODOPHYLLUM: When the rectum comes out of anus, prolapsus.
- ARS, CAUSTICUM, PHOS., NIT. ACID and MERC. SOL. should also be studied.

PROLAPSUS ANI

The last portion of our intestines sometimes comes out of the anal opening. It happens frequently in children but is found in adults also. The portion that comes out at the time of stools goes in of itself, but if it does not go in, it does so on pressing gently with the hand or linen. It occurs in constipation, diarrhoea, piles or dysentery and is cured with the original disease.

- PODOPHYLLUM: The chief remedy.
- ALOE: When urging of stools is uncontrollable and this happens after taking food.
- IGNATIA: When there is itching in anus.
- FERRUM PHOS.: For children.
- NUX VOM., LYCO., RATANHIA and PHOS. are also indicated.

HERNIA

When the intestines descend from the abdomen down to the scrotum, it is termed hernia. The belt is essential to check it.

- NUX VOM.: For left sided hernia, accompanied by constipation.
- LYCO.: For right sided hernia.
- LACHESIS: For left sided hernia.
- BELLADONNA: When there is pain around navel.
- SULPHURIC ACID, CALC. CARB. and SILICIA are also advised.

FISTULA

When an abscess in the rectum adopts chronic form, it is termed as fistula. When pus collects, there is swelling, it opens and pus is drained. This process is repeated again and again.

- BELLADONNA: When the abscess forms.
- MERCURIUS VIVUS: After the opening of the abscess.
- HEPAR SULPH. 3X TRIT.: This medicine hastens suppuration. 200 and higher potencies heal and prevent recurrence. The same is the case with SILICEA, in 1,000 and higher potencies it cures.
- CALCAREA SULPH. 6X, 200: May be used after the opening of the abscess to dry it up and heal.
- CALC. FLUOR., NITRIC ACID AND GRAPHITES are also indicated.

FISSURES

In this malady there are cracks at the anal opening, blood oozes out of them, but they are very painful, specially after stools.

- GRAPHITES: The chief remedy. When there is constipation, long lasting pain after passing stools.

- RATANHIA Q: When there are loose stools, burning, bleeding and severe pain as if broken glass pieces were there in the rectum, lasting long after stools.
- HAMAMELIS Q: When there is no pain but bleeding.
- AESCULUS: When the patient has piles, constipation, burning, ulcers.

WORMS

Worms are of several types. Generally small worms pass with stools and are not even an inch in length. Another type is round worms, two to four inches in length. Still another type is tape worms, several inches long.

- CINA: The chief remedy for all types of worms. Give it when the child is ever hungry and craves for sweets.
- STANNUM: This too is very efficacious.
- TEUCRIUM Q: When there is itching and burning at anus. For small worms.
- SANTONINE 3X TRIT.: When there is a biting sensation at anus and pain in abdomen. Give 2-3 times daily for several days.
- CHENOPODIUM OIL: For round worms give 10 drops with hot water 3 times daily.

Some physicians say that to destroy all sorts of worms give LYCO 30 for 2 days, then VERATRUM A.12 for 4 days, followed by IPECAC 6 for a week. Two doses daily may be given. Salt water should be syringed in the rectum in acute cases.

Tape worms are killed and expelled by the following mixture, 10 drops, in little water taken three times daily.:

- Potassium Iodide 35 grains
- Iodine 4 grains
- Distilled Water 1 ounce.

LIVER DISEASES

The liver is located on the right side of our abdomen and is a very important organ of our body. It produces bile, which digests our food. The main diseases of the liver are its enlargement, its inflammation, its cirrhosis, i.e., hardening, and jaundice (yellow eyes, urine and body). The following medicines have proved very efficacious in liver diseases.

- ACONITE: In acute cases when the patient has fever, pain, chill, jaundice, restlessness and fear.
- BRYONIA: In chronic cases when the patient has enlarged hard liver, constipation, sticking pain, vertigo, thirst, pain in the right shoulder, yellow eyes. Relief by lying on the right side.
- MERCURIUS: When the patient has jaundice, pain, which gets worse by lying on the right side. Useful both in acute and chronic cases.
- CHELIDONIUM Q, 30: When the patient has pain below right scapula. jaundice, diarrhoea or constipation.
- CHINA: When the patient has enlarged liver and spleen after a long lasting fever.
- NUX VOM.: In liver diseases due to drinking.
- LYCOPODIUM: Very efficacious in cirrhosis. When there is pain in the right axilla, flatulence, dark urine, the patient gets worse about 4-8 p.m.
- ARSENIC A.: When there is much thirst, swelling on face, hands and feet, burning and restlessness.
- LEPTANDRA: When the patient has black stools, swelling, jaundice, fluid in abdomen (dropsy).

INFANTILE LIVER

The liver of a new-born child is sufficiently enlarged but it shrinks gradually and drops below the ribs within a month or two. Sometimes this natural process is retarded and the liver remains enlarged. It is termed as Infantile Liver and is difficult to cure.

- CALCAREA ARS 3X TRIT.: 2-3 times daily dry on tongue. Very efficacious in these cases. It can be given with other indicated remedies. CALC., CARB. and LYCO. should also be studied in cases of infantile liver.
- MYRICA Q: 2 drops in water twice or thrice daily for jaundice.
- NATRUM MUR.: When fever gets worse from 11 a.m. to 5p.m., pain in liver, flatulence.
- NATRUM SULPH.: When there is pain in liver on breathing deeply, pain in abdomen on empty stomach which is relieved by eating something.
- CARDUUS Q: 2 to 5 drops with a little water 2-3 times daily for all liver troubles.
- BERBERIS V. Q: When there is pain in the gall bladder, bitter taste.
- HYDRASTIS Q: Useful in liver cases when there is constipation and jaundice.

ENLARGEMENT OF SPLEEN

Opposite to liver on the left side we have an organ called spleen. It is enlarged and becomes hard after long lasting fevers.

- CEANOTHUS Q: The chief remedy. 2-3 drops of mother tincture should be given 2-3 times daily. It covers nearly all symptoms of splenitis.
- ARSENIC, NATRUM MUR., CHINA and CARDUUS are also indicated in this disease.

10

DISORDERS OF THE HEAD AND FACE

HEADACHES

Headache is a very common symptom in many diseases, such as fevers, indigestion, lung diseases, rheumatism, etc., and the headache is gone when these diseases are cured. But sometimes headache appears all by itself, without any other disease whatsoever. The probable causes of a simple headache are cold, heat, loss of sleep, worry or tiresomeness. According to symptoms the following medicines may be given.

- BELLADONNA: Severe headache, aversion to light; eyes and face red; pain increases on lying, specially on the right side. Sudden attack after getting a haircut.
- ACONITE: Pain caused by sun or dry cold wind. Severe headache in half or the whole of the head. Feverish.
- BRYONIA: Pain in half of the head, specially at night. Increases with least motion. Bilious headache, bursting headache, vertigo, bitter vomiting. A peculiar symptom of this remedy is that pains begin from the front and are sticking, jerking and spread from the front to the back of the head, neck and in between shoulders.
- SPIGELIA: Pain on the left half side. It increases and

decreases with the sun, no pain after sunset. Pain travels from back to front.

- SANGUINARIA: Sun headache on the right side, relief from lying and rest.
- GLONOINE: Pain due to excessive heat or sun. Hemicrania.
- PULSATILLA: Pain due to indigestion or heavy fatty foods.
- NUX VOM.: Sun headache specially on the right side.
- PHOSPHORIC ACID: Pain due to excessive sexual indulgence.
- CHINA: Pain due to loss of semen or weakness caused by loss of blood or any vital fluid from the body.
- MAG. PHOS.: 5 tablets of 6x potency with hot water will often relieve ordinary headache.
- GELSEMIUM: Dull pain, heaviness, pain in temples, vertigo.
- MELILOTUS: Sick headache relieved by nose bleed or menses. Eyes heavy.

In addition to these medicines, head symptoms will be found almost in all the remedies. For Hemicrania of left side please also study THUJA, LACHESIS, CYCLAMEN and for the right side see PRUNUS SPINOSA, PLATINA, PULSATILLA and SILICIA.

TONSILLITIS

Tonsils become inflamed or enlarged mostly in children. Often removal by operation is advised. It is said that their function is not clear. In fact, they are watchdogs, protectors of lungs from infection. They become inflamed and thus prevent the infection going to lungs. Often there is pain in the throat, which increases on swallowing and slight fever occurs. In chronic cases there are ulcers on tonsils and they become septic, that is, pus is formed in them. Homoeopathic medicines help to avoid the operation.

- BELLADONNA: In acute cases when the right side is affected, even liquids are swallowed with difficulty, tonsils are inflamed.

- MERC SOL.: This is used after BELLADONNA. When there is profuse salivation, and signs of pus.
- MERC IOD RUB 3X TRIT.: For left sided tonsillitis. Pain increases in the night, the patient is better in day time.
- MERC IOD FLAV 3X TRIT.: When the right side is affected and there is nightly aggravation. Both these medicines should be given 3-4 grains dry on tongue. No liquid drink for half an hour. Keep the medicines well covered, they are spoiled by light and sun.
- CALCAREA FLUOR. 6X: When the tonsils are stony hard.
- CALCAREA PHOS. 6X, KALI MUR 6X and FERRUM PHOS. 6X: These three medicines are useful in all the stages. They can be given singly or all the three combined with a little hot water. Gargles with warm salt water are very useful.
- LUTEINUM: 200 or 1000 should be given inter-currently with other medicines once a week or a month.
- AGRAPHIS NUTANS Q: When adenoids are also enlarged with tonsils, this is the best medicine. One drop of Q may be given 2-3 times daily for some time. In adenoid growth the nose is obstructed, the child breathes with the mouth and sleeps with his mouth open. This medicine can be used in 3X or 6X also.
- TUBERCULINUM: A weekly dose of 200 potency in chronic cases.
- SULPHUR, CALCAREA CARB., HEPAR and BACILLINUM should also be thought of, sour and cold things like iced water or ice cream etc. should be avoided.

SPEECH PROBLEMS

- CUPRUM MET.: When there is speech difficulty due to spasm in throat.
- AGARICUS: When the spasm is in the tongue.
- STRAMONIUM: For stammering, inarticulate, slow and difficult speech.

- STANNUM: When there is difficulty due to debility of the chest.
- LACHESIS: When there is a complete loss of speech and the tongue does not come out of the mouth.
- HYOSCYAMUS: For loss of speech due to fear.
- CAUSTICUM: For loss of speech or hoarseness due to paralysis of vocal cords.

DISEASES OF THE EYES

CONJUNCTIVITIS

Inflammation of the conjunctiva of the eyes.

- FERUM PHOS. 6X: 5 tablets or 5 grains dissolved in hot water 3-4 times a day will subside ordinary inflammation, pain or redness of eyes.
- BELLADONNA: Pain in eyes, eyes red, the patient does not like light and heat.
- ACONITE: Pain due to cold or dry cold winds.
- MERC. COR.: Pus in eyes, eyelids stick together.
- APIS. MEL.: Eyelids swollen, stinging pain, pus, itching.
- EUPHRASIA: Excessive discharge of water from eyes and nose, red eyes, light unbearable. Mother tincture of EUPHRASIA be mixed with rose water or distilled water in proportion of 1 to 10 and used as eye lotion, two or three times a day. Eyes be formented with hot BORIC LOTION (BORIC ACID 1, hot water 10). Washing of eyes with cold water in which Triphala is soaked overnight is very sedative. Mud plaster on eyes is also recommended.

NIGHT-BLINDNESS

- PHYSOSTIGMA: is the head remedy for this diseases.
- BELLADONNA and NUX: These are also used according to

symptoms. This happens due to the lack of Vitamin A. Butter with sugar candy and black pepper should be taken. This alone has cured night-blindness.

DAY-BLINDNESS

Sees well in the night but nothing during the day.

- BOTHROPS: is the chief remedy.
- LYCO., PHOS. and RANUNCULUS may also be studied.

PARTIAL BLINDNESS

- AURUM MET.: When the patient sees only the upper half of an object.
- LITHIUM CARB.: When the patient sees only the left half of an object.
- LYCO.: When the patient does not see the right half.
- TITANIUM: When only half of an object is seen. The patient feels giddy, has imperfect vision.
- NATRUM MUR., SEPIA and CALCAREA CARB. should also be studied.

STYES

PULSATILLA, HEPAR, STAPHYSAGRIA, MERC. SOL., SULPHUR, CAUSTICUM and ALUMINA are indicated when styles appear on upper eyelids. ASTERIAS, PHOS. and RHUS TOX. for lower lids. LYCO. and STANNUM when the eruptions are in the corner of lids.

- HEPAR: When pus is formed.
- MERC SOL.: When styes are repeated, 200 should be tried once a week or so.

CATARACT

It is a common disease in India. In old age the lenses of the eyes gradually become dim and eyesight is effected. When a lens becomes completely opaque, it is removed by operation, a fluid takes its place and suitable glasses are given to restore eyesight. If cataract is detected in its early stages, it is often cured or its progress is retarded by suitable Homoeopathic medicines. In the early stages the vision becomes clouded and often the patient sees better in twilight and is worse during sunshine. Dr. Burnelt of London has claimed to have cured cases without operation.

- SULPHUR: 200 or of high potency should be given once a week or even fortnightly. If there is a history of suppression of some skin disease, this remedy suits. In cases, where cataract starts in the right eye and then it effects the left, this remedy is successful.
- PHOSPHORUS: Dim vision, black spots before the eyes, the patient sees better on shading the eyes with his hand or some book or cardboard. A green halo around light. High and higher potencies at longer intervals.
- CALCAREA FLUOR 6X or 12X: This is the chief remedy; should be used continuously for months. 4 or 5 tablets twice daily.
- CAUSTICUM: The patient wants to rub eyes frequently. Black spots.
- LYCOPODIUM: It has been successfully used in cases which resulted after suppression of menses or after a long lasting fever.

NATRUM MUR., SEPIA, SILICEA, EUPHRASIA should also be studied. Treatment should be continued for at least 6 to 12 months. SUCCUS CINERARIA MARITIMA, one or two drops 2-3 times daily should be dropped in eyes. Eyes should be washed well with cold water in the morning.

LOSS OF VISION

Sometimes suddenly eyesight becomes dim. It may be due to looking long at the shining sun or a bright light. It may also be the result of taking wines or narcotics, or due to chill or suppression of sweats or menses, or excessive bleeding.

- CHINA 6 or 30: Two doses daily for some time, if due to bleeding, etc.
- PHOSPHORUS: According to its symptoms.
- NUX VOM.: When due to excessive drinking.
- BELLADONNA: Red face, infected eyes, rush of blood to head.
- PULSATILLA: When due to suppressed menses. Exposure to sun should be avoided. Bright light or sun effects vision.

SQUINTING

- ALUMINA is the chief remedy.
- SPIGELIA and CINA when there is a history of worms.
- HYOSCYAMUS, GELS and STRAMONIUM should also be studied.

GRANULAR EYES

- EUPHRASIA: Watery eyes, pus in eyes, pain in eyelids. Lotion of its mother tincture in proportion of 1 to 10 of rose water or distilled water should be used as eye drops 2-3 times a day. Boil neem leaves and wash the eyes with its water.
- ARGENTUM NIT.: When the granules are troublesome.
- AURUM: Hot water in eyes, the patient dislikes light, has dim vision.

- NATRUM MUR.: Heat and sun increases the trouble. Profuse watering of eyes.
- PULSATILLA: Tears in eyes, cold air gives relief, trouble increases during evening.
- THUJA: When the granules are bigger in size.

LACHRYMAL FISTULA

There is a tube-like duct which runs from the inner corner of the eyes to inner nose, and is called lachrymal duct. Sometimes pus is formed and fistula results in this duct. It sometimes recurs even after operation.

- SILICEA 1000: Once a week often cures this fistulous ulcer.
- FLOURIC ACID: The second best remedy,

CALCAREA CARB, HEPAR, NATRUM MUR., PETROLEUM, PULSATILLA and SULPHUR are also indicated.

DISEASES OF THE EARS

EARACHE (OTITIS)

There are many causes of pain in the ears. Exposure to cold wind or severe cold, injury, suppression of skin disease, boil in the ear, inflammation of the ear, deposit of ear wax etc. may produce sticking or stinging pain and may result in formation of a boil in which pus may be formed. After suppuration, i.e., pus formation, pain is relieved and the ear begins to discharge pus.

- ACONITE: Pain due to cold.
- BELLADONNA: Sudden pain accompanied by headache. Inflammation or boil in the ear.
- PULSATILLA: Lancinating pain. Pain in children after measles.
- APIS: Stinging pain.

- MERC SOL.: After small-pox, pain extends to the teeth and increases at night on sleeping on a warm bed. Formation of pus.
- CHAMOMILLA: Pain in teeth also. In children pain during dentition.
- ARNICA: Pain due to injury.
- SILICEA: Pus, offensive odour.
- HEPAR: Pain after pus is formed.

Ear should be washed with a lotion of PLANTAGO Q, 20 drop for one ounce of hot water. Put 2-3 drops of BELLADONNA GLYCERINE (BELL Q 1 part, GLYCERINE 10 parts) in the ear and then cover with cotton.

- HEPAR and SILICEA: In high potencies (200-1000) once a week or so are very useful in chronic ottorrhoea (discharge of pus).

TELLURIUM, MERC. SOL., NITRIC ACID and CALC. CARB. should also be studied for chronic otorrhoea.

In offensive discharge the ear should be washed with carbolic lotion. Take CARBOLIC ACID 1 dram, GLYCERINE 1 ounce, distilled water 5 ounces and mix well. Ear should not be washed too much and frequently. In the night blow a few grains of BORIC ACID into the ear and wash with simple hot water in the morning. This will reduce the discharge.

DEAFNESS

There is no remedy for those who are deaf and dumb since birth but when a person becomes total or partly deaf due to weakness of nerves or any other cause, he can be cured or relieved by suitable medicines.

- PHOSPHORUS: The head remedy in all sorts of deafness.

Often deafness occurs after typhoid, and if so, this remedy will cure it. When there is roaring or ringing in the ear, or echoing.

- CHINA: When deafness is due to a loss of vital fluids from the body. When there is ringing in the ears.
- ACID PHOS: When it is due to sexual indulgences.

GRAPHITES, SULPHUR, SILICEA and DULCAMARA should also be studied.

RINGING

There are different sorts of sounds in the ears — ringing, roaring, hissing, buzzing, etc.

- THIOSINAMINUM: In all sorts of sounds.

ACID PHOS, CHINA, CHIN. SULPH., DIGITALIS, BELLADONNA should also be considered.

ECZEMA

This disease can affect any part of the body, but quite often it attacks the back of the ear, external ear or even internal ear. There is severe itching and oozing of sticky fluid and sometimes pus is formed.

- GRAPHITES: The head remedy in all sorts of eczemas.
- RHUS TOX.: When there are blisters in and around.
- ARSENIC A. and SULPHUR: In chronic cases.
- MEZEREUM: When the patient thrusts his finger in the ear frequently and feels as if cold air was entering the ear.
- PETROLEUM: When it increases during winter and subsides in summer. When there is pain on touching the ear, itch and sounds in ears.

- PSORINUM: In chronic cases when it increases during winter. 200 or 1000 once a week or month.

NOSE DISEASES

COLD AND CATARRH

Cold is a disease of very common occurrence. When there is inflammation of the mucus membrane of the nose, a watery discharge comes out after 2 to 3 days. This discharge becomes thick and eventually it disappears. Though cold and catarrh is often confined to the nose, the disease affects the whole body. The patient feels pain all over the body, sometimes the temperature also rises a little, and cough is often accompanied and persists even after the catarrh is suspended. Sometimes the inflammation of the mucus membrane of the nose extends to the lungs and may turn into bronchitis or pneumonia.

Some are of the opinion that simple cold should be carefully treated as it may be the precursor of many serious diseases. Scientists believe that cold is contagious like other such diseases.

Though the immediate cause is getting chilled, taking bath after perspiration, a sudden change of temperature, getting wet in rains, going out in dry cold winds, etc., but the real cause is indigestion. If a man's digestion is not impared, and there is no overeating, he will not catch cold even when exposed to cold winds, etc. Whenever one has cold, a light diet should be taken. Fasting for a day or two or taking only of a liquid diet will soon cure the catarrh. Homoeopathic medicines are very useful in this disease. Hot water should be sipped during an attack.

- SPIRIT CAMPHOR: In the beginning stage, when there is a sensation of cold in the body. When there is yawning and a bruised feeling all over, 2 or 3 drops of mother tincture should be taken in sugar or sugar of milk every one or two hours. Often the attack is thus cut short. If one has to go out in severe cold 4-5 drops of CAMPHOR may be taken with sugar. It will act as a prophylactic and will protect one from catching cold.

- FERUM PHOS. 6X: About 5 grains of powder or 5 tablets should be taken, dissolved in half a cup of hot water, every 2 or 3 hours for 2 or 3 days.
- ACONITE 3X or 30: In the first stage when there is a little fever and sneezing, bruised feeling and chilliness, after exposure to dry cold winds.
- DULCAMARA: When the cold is due to wet atmosphere, in the rainy season.
- NATRUM SULPH.: When it is due to getting wet or taking a bath.
- NATRUM MUR.: Watery discharge from nose and eyes, sneezing, etc.
- ALLIUM CEPA: Watery acid discharge, the patient feels better in open air.
- GELSEMIUM: Catarrh during summer season, the patient wants to lie down with closed eyes. Heaviness in head, chill in back.
- ARSENIC: Restlessness, thirst but the patient drinks little, watery burning discharge, extreme prostration.
- PULSATILLA: In the second and third stage of cattarh, when the discharge becomes thick and yellowish, the patient feels worse in a closed room and in the evening.
- NUX VOMICA: When there is constipation, one nostril is stopped, watery discharge during the day, but the nose is stopped in open air and during night.
- SAMBUCUS: When there is stoppage of nose in children.
- KALI BICHROM.: During the later stage when the discharge is sticky and ropy.
- MERC. SOL.: When there is pain in throat and nose, yellowish discharge, the patient feels cold and hot alternately.
- MERC COR.: Much sneezing, ulcers in nose.

- AMMONIUM CARB.: Stoppage of nose in the night, specially in children. Cough at about 3 or 4 a.m.
- BRYONIA: When the cold is extended to chest, there is stinging pain in chest, cough troublesome. Cough is excited when the patient comes in a closed room from outside.
- SILICIA: Old catarrh when the discharge is pus like.

Gargles with hot salted water are always useful in cold.

OZAENA

In this disease there are ulcers in the mucus membrane of the nose, offensive pus is discharged, and even necrosis of bone sets in.

- CADMIUM SULPH.: The chief remedy. 3X powder two or three times daily should be taken for a sufficiently long time.
- AURUM MET.: Pain and heat in the nose, yellowish offensive discharge.
- KALI BICHROM.: When middle of the nose becomes depressed, discharge is offensive, mixed with pus and blood.
- ACID NITRIC: When the disease is caused by abuse of mercury or its compounds.
- ARS, SYPH, and PULS should be also studied.

EPISTAXIS

Bleeding from nose.

- FERRUM IODATUM: This is the head remedy. 3x powder 2-3 grains twice or thrice daily on the tongue.
- MILLEFOLIUM: 2-3 drops of mother tincture 2-3 times daily with water will stop bleeding specially of red blood.

- AMBRA GRISEA: Particularly useful for bilious patients.
- HAMAMELIS: Mother tincture 2-3 drops in water will stop dark or clotted blood. Give 30 or 200 to avoid recurrence.
- ARNICA: Nose bleed due to injury.
- TRILLIUM: When there is deep red thick blood, apply mother tincture externally in the nose, it will stop bleeding. 3 to 6 potency be given internally.
- CHINA: Bleeding due to debility or debility due to bleeding.
- VIPERA: Very useful in chronic complaints. 30 or 200 be given weekly.
- FERRUM PIC. 3X, SULPHUR, LACHESIS and NUX VOM. are also indicated sometimes.

POLYPUS

Often there is a fleshy growth in one or both the nostrils. It is soft and smooth. It is removed by operation but reappears after some time. The following Homoeopathic remedies will cure it.

- FORMICA RUFA 1X: Twice daily is very useful.
- THUJA: 200 be given weekly and Q to be applied externally on the growth.
- PHOS.: When the polypus bleeds. 30 to 200 weekly.
- SANGUINARIA NIT. 1X: Use internally twice daily and apply the powder externally also.

TEETH PROBLEMS

ODONTALGIA

Pain in teeth.

- PLANTAGO: 30 or 200 internally and Q to be applied externally in the affected tooth. Cotton saturated with PLANTAGO Q should be put over the painful tooth.

- CAMPHOR Q: Apply externally cotton saturated with Q.
- POTASSIUM PERMANG.: Dissolve 3-4 grains in a glass of water and gargle twice or thrice daily.
- NUX VOM.: When cold water increases the pain or it is due to overuse of coffee or wine.
- CHAMOMILLA, BRYONIA and ANTIM CRUD.: When hot water increases the pain.
- MAGNESIA PHOS. 3X or 6X: Dissolved in hot water will often relieve pain; may be repeated every half hour.
- MERC. SOL.: When cold as well as hot water increases the pain. Pain increases in the night, much salivation or pus in gums.
- PHOS.: For bleeding gums.
- PULS.: When pain is relieved by cold water and increases by hot drinks.
- ACONITE, BELLADONNA and NUX: Useful when pain is due to exposure to cold during winter.
- KREOSOTE: For decayed teeth.
- STAPHYSAGRIA: When teeth become black, pain increases with cold food or drink or air.
- BRYONIA: When pain increases by smoking or taking hot drinks or food. Teeth seem elongated.
- NATRUM MUR.: When pain occurs from 10-11 a.m. to 4-5 p.m.
- SILICIA: When gums are swollen or there is a gum boil, or pus in gums.
- CARBO VEG.: When the gums are bleeding or receding, pain increases by taking cold, hot or saltish things.
- HEKLA LAVA: When there is abscess in gums, the jaw is swollen, difficult teething.
- ANTIM CRUD.: When there is pain on taking sour food or drink.
- SEPIA: When pain increases from 6 to 12 a.m. and on lying down.
- CALCAREA FLUOR.: When there are sores on teeth, deficiency of calcium. 6X twice daily.

- HEPAR SULPH.: When pain increases with cold, there is pain in the root of the teeth or abscess in teeth. Begin with 3x, when pus comes out give 30 to 200.

ABCESS OR ULCER IN GUMS

- BELLADONNA: If taken in the beginning its use may subside the abscess.
- MERC SOL.: When pus is formed, give 3x or 6x twice or thrice daily.
- HEPAR SULPH.: Begin with 3x, when pus comes out 30 or 200 will dry it up.
- CALCAREA SULPH.: Very effective for drying up the abscess after the boil bursts.
- SILICIA: It will bring out pus and heal up the wounds. Strengthens teeth. Cold aggravates, it heat ameliorates.

PYORRHOEA

In this disease the ulcers of the gums become chronic and though there is little pain, pus oozes out of them. This pus is swallowed which impairs digestion. The pus is often offensive. Many persons have to get all their teeth extracted because of pyorrhoea but if care is taken in the beginning and medicine is used the disease can be cured. Often a hard brush produces pyorrhoea, soft brush or *datun* of neem should be used. Rubbing the gums with mustard oil mixed with salt is very useful.

- HEPAR SULPH.: 3x should be used for chilly patients. If the disease is chronic, 200 or higher potencies should be used.
- SILICEA: For chilly but lean and thin patients 200 or higher potencies.
- MERC SOL.: 30 or 200 when there is salivation and profuse pus.

- NITRIC ACID: If the cause of the disease is abuse of mercury.
- CALENDULA Q: For gargles 3 or 4 times a day, one part mixed with ten parts of lukewarm water.

FISTULA

Sometimes the gum abscess becomes chronic and turns into fistula.

- SILICEA: 30, 200, 1000 is the head remedy.
- FLOURIC ACID: In chronic cases, higher potencies work well.

FACE PROBLEMS

ACNE

A skin condition characterized by red pimples on the skin, especially on the face, due to inflamed or infected sebaceous glands and prevalent chiefly among adolescents. Popularly called Puberty Boils.

- KALI BROM.: Chief remedy. Should be used for sometime in 6 to 30 potency.
- ASTERIAS ERUBENS: When there are red pimples on the side of the nose, chin and mouth. Disposition to pimples of adolescence.
- RADIUM BROMIDE: In 30 potency if the above two remedies do not work.
- BERBERIS AQUIFOLIUM Q: 2 drops twice daily. Specially effective in case of girls.
- DULCAMARA: If the pimples appear before menses.
- ARS 1000 and SULPHUR IODIDE 3X TRIT.: When the number of pimples is quite large and they are hard and do not burst and pus does not come out of them. 2-3 grains

should be given dry on tongue. Keep the power covered, it is decomposed from light.

- BORAX 3X, ACID NIT. and GRAPHITES should also be studied.

CHIN-ITCHING

Sometimes small boils or pimples on the chin itch and pus is also formed.

- RHUS TOX.: The chief remedy.
- SULPHUR: If itch extends tear the nose and eyes.
- GRAPHITES: If it is eczema-like, with sticky discharge, and gives a feeling as if there was a cobweb on the face.
- LYCOPODIUM: For bleeding ulcers, scaly or scabby eruptions.

UNWANTED HAIR

Sometimes hair grows on the face of women due to overactivity of some glands. THUJA, LYCO, NAT. MUR., PHOS. and THYROIDINUM are some important remedies. These may be tried according to the symptoms and nature of the patient.

LIPS

- CONDURANGO: For cracks in lips, ulcers in corners of the mouth. Very effective even for cancer of mouth or lips.
- NAT. MUR.: For itching, cracks, blisters, cancer.
- CONIUM, HYDRASTIS, SEPIA and ARS. A. are some useful remedies for the cancer of lips.

NEURALGIA OF FACE

A severe sharp pain felt along the length of a nerve, especially in the head or face.

- ACONITE: When there is pain and tingling.
- MEZEREUM: When the pain is aggravated after taking food and ameliorated by heat.
- BELLADONNA: When there is sudden pain on the right side which subsides also suddenly.
- CHAMOMILLA: When there is severe pain which extends to neck, teeth and ears.
- SYPHILINUM: For pain which increases in the night.

PARALYSIS OF THE FACE

It is often on the half side of the face, lips hang down on one side, speech is impaired, one eye hangs down.

- ACONITE: When due to exposure to dry cold.
- CAUSTICUM: When it is on the right side due to exposure to cold air.
- GRAPHITES: When the patient feels, as if there is a cobweb on the face.
- ALUMINA: When the patient feels as if the white of an egg or blood has dried on the face.
- BELLADONNA: When it is on the right side.
- CADMIUM SULPH. and SENEGA Q: For the left side.
- PTYALISM: When there is profuse salivation and a watery discharge from the mouth.
- MERC SOL.: The chief remedy.
- NATRUM MUR. and PULS. are also used according to symptoms.

TONGUE DISEASES

ULCERS

The tongue becomes red or inflamed due to indigestion and often small ulcers are formed which are painful.

- BORAX 6X: When these ulcers are whitish.
- FERRUM PHOS 6X: For red and inflamed tongue.
- MERC SOL.: When accompanied by watery secretion from the mouth.
- ARUM TRIPH.: When there are cracks and blood oozes out of them.
- CANTHARIS: When the tongue is inflamed due to some hot drink or food.

CANCER IN TONGUE

- KALI ÇYANATUM: This medicine has arrested and cured many cases of tongue cancer. Use it when there is agonising pain.
- PHOSPHORUS: When the patient wants to drink ice cold water and the pain and irritation is relieved by drinking it.
- AURUM MET., CONDURANGO, CONIUM, CALCAREA FLUOR., THUJA, ARS. A. and APIS should also be studied.

THICK WHITE COATING

This is the chief symptom of ANTIM. CRUDUM and KALI MUR. The tongue of ARS. is dry and that of IPECAC red.

11

SKIN DISEASES

ITCH (PRURITIS)

This is a common complaint. External ointments, oils or lotions should not be used. They suppress the itch and the suppression affects the internal organs of the body and causes many serious complaints. A hot wash with boiled neem leaves is advised. Soaps should be avoided.

- SULPHUR: When there is burning after itching, it gets worse on washing or at night or from heat. Recurs in spring and damp weather, unhealthy skin, every little injury suppurates.
- FAGOPYRUM: When there is much itching, it gets better by washing with cold water and worse on scratching, touch and retiring and in sunlight.
- MEZEREUM: When there is uncontrollable itching, so much so that blood comes out.
- DULCIS: When there is intense itching and the patient scratches it with brush or rubs his back with the trunk of a tree or wall.
- PSORINUM: In chronic cases.

- BELLADONNA: When the skin is red but itch is less.
- RHUS TOX.: When there are vesicles, intense itching, parts red and swollen, gets worse in cold and better in heat.
- RADIUM BROM. 30: Once a week only. To be taken when skin becomes colourless after itch, or there is itch in anus or bleeding after itch.
- ARS: When there is intense burning, restlessness and anguish.
- APIS: When there is swelling, stinging pain, itch gets worse with heat.
- AMBRA GRISEA: When there is intense itching on the genitals of men and women, worse on testicles.
- OLEANDER: When there is itch on the head of children, gets worse with cold.
- SEPIA: When there are round red patches at the itching spot, too many on elbows and knees, get worse with cold air, washing, after sweating.
- TUBERCULINUM: When other remedies fail, give one dose of this in 7 to 15 days.
- SPONGIA Q: Useful in almost all skin diseases. 2 drops twice daily.
- ACID CARBOLIC: When there are water eruptions all over with itch.
- SARSAPARILLA: When the itch is worse during morning and evening, and there are pimples after itching.

BOILS AND ABSCESSES

- ACONITE: When swelling is accompanied with fever.
- BELLADONNA: When the swelling is red and painful.
- MERC SOL.: When there is a tendency to pus.
- APIS: When there is itching, pain and swelling
- HEPAR S. 3X: It will hasten suppuration and relieve the pain, the boil will burst open. Give 200 after the boil opens and pus is expelled.

- SILICEA 6X: For hastening the abscess and opening it. Give 200, 1000 to dry up pus and heal chronic cases.
- ARNICA: When there are crops of small boils.
- CALCAREA SULPH. 6X: After the opening of the abscess it will hasten healing.
- FLUORIC ACID: When the ulcer becomes fistulous—in rectum, eyes or nose.
- MERC. VIVUS: When there is abscess in the root of tooth.
- PYROGEN: A tendency to boils, pus offensive.
- ARS: For gangrenes.
- ECHINACEA Q: Has cured chronic gangrenes. 5 drops twice daily. Dress with its 1-10 lotion.
- CALENDULA Q: To be taken internally thrice daily. Its ointment is very useful for healing up ulcers.

ECZEMA

- GRAPHITES: Head remedy, useful both in dry and wet cases. Use when skin becomes thick. Most chronic cases have been cured by a few doses of 200 or 1000 given at long intervals.
- PSORINUM: For old cases. When there are ulcers, offensive pus, intense itching, use 200 or 1000 infrequently.
- RHUS VEN. and RHUS TOX.: When there is intense itching, with vesicular eruptions. Formation of scales. 200 or 1000 at long intervals.
- CICUTA V.: For eczema of hairy parts, specially chin. For itch-less eczema, which dries into hard crusts.
- CROTON: For eczema of face, genitals, scrotum, when there is much itching.
- OLEANDER: When it is wet on scalp, pus turns into hard crusts, on itching pus or fluid oozes out.
- KALI MUR.: For all sorts of eczema in which whitish scaly crusts are formed. When eczema is due to after effects of

vaccination, in ladies due to scanty menses or amenorrhoea, on the face and head of children.

- HEPAR S.: When it is specially on scrotum, gets worse with cold. Pus.
- BOVISTA: When it is on the back of the hands, wet in the bends of the knees, gets worse on full moon.
- TUBERCULINUM: 200, 1000 once a month or so in chronic obstinate cases. Thick skin, black colour. Use when well selected remedies fail.
- SULPHUR: When there is intense burning and itching, red orifices, offensive odor from body.
- ALUMINA: When it is dry, scaly, on the scalp and face, crusts over scalp, thin, foetid, excoriating discharge.
- PETROLEUM: When it is dry, scaly, appearing in winter on hands and behind the ears.
- MEZEREUM, ARS, THUJA, CLEMATIS, AGARICUS, ANTIM. CRUD. should also be studied.

RINGWORM

This is a well known disease in which there is great itching. External ointments made from hrysophanic Acid are extensively used. It is said that the worms are destroyed by it. 4 gms. of CHRYSOPHANIC ACID mixed with one ounce of olive oil is applied on ringworms.

- BACILLINUM 200: Once a week for old cases.
- LYCO and GRAPHITES: When it is outside the upper lips and there is dryness.
- NATRUM SULPH. 200: Once a week.
- ANTIM. CRUD.: When it is near the nails or on mustaches.
- HEPAR: When it is on private parts, gets worse with cold or in winter.
- TELLURIUM: When it is on chin, has offensive discharge. Other medicines mentioned under eczema will also be useful.

CORNS

A small, painful area of thickened skin on the foot, especially on the toes, caused by pressure.

- FERRUM PICRICUM 3X: Chief remedy for corns.
- NITRIC ACID: When there is pus and burning.
- GRAPHITES, RANUNCULUS B. and THUJA should be studied. HYDRASTIS Q mixed with glycerine or oil should be applied externally.

CARBUNCLE

This is an abscess which tends to turn into gangrene. It is mostly seen in diabetic patients. Treatment of diabetes will be necessary to cure it.

- ANTHRACINUM 30, 200: If given at the beginning, will cure it.
- APIS MEL.: When there is stinging pain.
- ARSENIC: When it gets septic.
- ECHINACEA: Has been curative in gangrenous carbuncles.
- TARENTULA C.: Relieves pain and tension.
- LACHESIS: When the ulcer becomes blue.

WARTS

Painless eruptions on any portion of the body (popularly known as *Massa* in Hindi).

- THUJA: Very successful remedy. 200 or 1000 infrequently for all kinds of warts.
- CAUSTICUM: When these are small in size all over the body, mostly on the face and hands.
- SABINA: For fig warts with intolerable itching and burning.

- NITRIC ACID: When warts are painful, moist, syphlitic.
- NAT. SULPH.: For general use to cure warts.
- BUFO: When there are on hands.
- CINNAB: When there is bleeding.
- FERRUM PIC., ANTIM. CRUD., CALC. C. and DULCAMARA are also indicated.

NETTLE-RASH (URTICARIA)

Red patch like eruptions all over the body with much itching and burning, appear suddenly and subside suddenly.

- CALCAREA CARB.: When rash disappears on slightest exposure or fresh air.
- RHUS TOX.: When these get worse during rains or cold weather or under cold air.
- ANTIM. CRUD.: When these get worse on washing and under heat or sun.
- APIS: When there is oedematous swelling, gets worse under heat, stinging pain.
- URTICA URENS: When there is vomiting and diarrhoea after suppression of eruptions.
- CHLORAL HYDRATE 3X: Should be given if the above remedies do not act.
- ASTACUS FL.: When these are due to liver disturbance.
- SKOOKUM-CHUCK 3, 6: When the patient has other skin diseases.
- ARS and SULPHUR: In chronic cases.

NAILS

- THUJA: For diseased and waxy nails.
- ARUM. TRI.: For biting of nails till they bleed.
- SILICEA: For ingrowing and deformed toe nalis.

- GRAPHITES: For thickened nails.
- CAUSTICUM: For ingrowing of nails after the use of SILICEA.
- ANTIM. CRUD.: For brittle and out of shape nails.

12

RESPIRATORY DISORDERS

HOARSENESS

There is a sound box (larynx) in the throat with which we speak. Due to cold, overuse of voice or any sudden atmospheric change, speech becomes hoarse and difficult on account of inflammation.

- ACONITE: When it is due to dry cold winds and there is dry cough, and fever.
- BELLADONNA: When the face is red, fever high, and the patient has a barking sound.
- SPONGIA: When there is pain and hoarseness. Is useful after ACONITE is given.
- CHENOPODIUM: When there is a complete loss of voice.
- HEPAR SULPH.: When there is cough, with phlegm, increases during cold, the patient gets relief from heat.
- LACHESIS: When there is aggravation from hot drinks, constriction, the patient wants to open the shirt buttons at the throat.
- KALI BICHROM.: When the phlegm is sticky, ropy and thick.
- CAUSTICUM: When the patient passes urine involuntarily while coughing.

- CUPRUM MET.: When there are cramps in the throat, constriction, pale face, suffocation, and fists are clinched.
- FERRUM PIC.: When there is hoarseness due to delivering a speech or overuse of voice. 3X TRIT. dry on the tongue 2-3 times will give relief.

BRONCHITIS (INFLAMMATION OF THE AIR TUBES)

The mucus membrane of the air tubes is inflamed due to cold, suppression of perspiration, etc., and fever, difficult breathing and cough are common symptoms. Sometimes it takes a serious turn, specially in children.

- ACONITE: If given early it will avert the attack.
- ANTIM TART.: 3X TRIT. is useful for children and old men when there is a rattling sound in the throat and chest and the patient cannot eject phlegm. Fever is not high, hands and feet are cold. Should be repeated 4-6 times a day.
- BRYONIA: When there is dry troublesome cough, pain in the chest which is relieved by pressing the chest. Bloody phlegm, cough is aggravated by entering a warm room and by motion.
- KALI BICHROM.: When there is very stingy, ropy, thick glutinous expectoration.
- PHOSPHORUS: When the patient cannot lie on his left side, the pain increases, he has cough by going out in the cold, and sweat, expectoration sometimes bloody. The medicine should not be repeated too often, one dose of 30 a day will be sufficient.
- LYCOPODIUM: When the right lung is attacked. This medicine follows well after ANTIM TART.
- HEPAR SULPH.: When there is aggravation from cold, cold air or cold drinks. In chronic cases. Yellowish phlegm.
- SULPHUR, BACILLINUM and TUBERCULINUM: Useful in old cases.

PLEURISY

When the covering membrane of the lungs is inflamed, it is termed pleurisy. There is severe pain in the chest, fever, cough, and sometimes a watery fluid collects between the lungs and membranes.

- ACONITE: Very useful in the beginning.
- BRYONIA: Follows well after ACONITE. BRYONIA is the chief remedy of the disease. There is burning in the chest, stinging pain, least motion aggravates it, and even deep breath is painful. There is dry cough, constipation and thirst.
- APIS MEL.: When fluid collects. There is stinging pain, the patient cannot lie on his left side. The patient does not feel thirsty.
- RANUNCULUS BULB.: This is an important remedy of this disease. There are adhesions of the mucus membranes sometimes, and there is great pain. It works well in adhesions and when the fluid collects.
- ARS. A.: In chronic cases. CANTHARIS, KALI CARB., PHOS., SILICEA, SULPHUR and ARNICA are some other remedies indicated in this disease and should also be considered.

PNEUMONIA

Inflammation of lungs is called pneumonia. High fever, difficult breathing, thirst and restlessness are the primary symptoms. In the second stage, exudation in lungs collects and comes out as sputum. In the third stage, sputum is ejected easily, fever subsides, and cough remains for some time. In bad cases, the third stage does not come and the disease takes a serious turn. Then the sputum increases, extremities get cold, temperature falls to subnormal and subsequently the patient expires. A physician should be consulted in this disease. However, the following medicines are found useful.

- ACONITE: Use it in the beginning.
- PHOS.: When the phlegm is rusty. The patient cannot lie on his left side.
- HEPAR: In chronic cases.
- BRYONIA: When the case is complicated with pleurisy.
- LYCO: When the right sided case is in its last stage, and there is fan-like motion of nostrils.
- ANTIM TART.: When there is cold sweating and a gurgling sound of sputum in the throat and in lungs. The patient has sub-normal temperature.
- VERATRUM VIR.: In the first stage, when there is congestion, in lungs and restlessness.
- SULPHUR, IODIUM, BACILL., CHELIDONIUM and ARS. A. are also used.

ASTHMA

Asthma is chronic bronchitis and is a tough disease. The spasm occurs in the muscles around the air tubes, and difficult breathing, cough etc. occurs. The patient cannot lie. Paroxysm or fits occur now and then.

During fit or attack ACONITE Q, IPECAC Q, LOBELIA Q, CUPRUM Q, NATRUM SULPH. 6X, ASPIDOSPERMA Q, SENEGA Q and MAGNESIA PHOS. 3X TRIT. have proved useful. They should be given in hot water.

- BLATTA ORIENTALIS Q: This medicine is often useful to the patients who have had malaria. 1 or 2 drops 3 times a day,
- BACILLINUM A.: When the attack is worse after midnight, the patient cannot lie, he has cold sweats, and thirsts for small quantities of water, and the attack subsides after 3 or 4 a.m.
- CARBO VEG.: When the patient sits and gasps for air as if he is hungry for air.

- IPECAC 1X or 3X: During the attack one drop hourly or half hourly subsides it.
- ARALIA Q or 6 or 30: When the attack comes after the first sleep at about 11-12 p.m. and there is dry coughing, which gets worse on lying, nasal catarrh, the patient feels as if there was something in the throat that chokes, also sneezing.
- NAT MUR., NAT SULPH., MAG. PHOS., KALI PHOS.: A mixture of all the four in 6X TRIT. should be given half hourly during the attack with hot water.
- ERIODICTYON Q: 5 to 20 drops of Q often subsides a severe attack, given hourly with hot water. After the fit it should be used in 6 potency once or twice daily. The patient sweats at night and expectoration gives him relief. Tubercular patients are benefited by this remedy.
- BACILLINUM or TUBERCULINUM: Once a week are useful in chronic cases.

COUGH

Cough is not a disease in itself; it occurs in many diseases of the lung and throat. However, a few medicines are quoted here.

- ACONITE: When it is due to cold and gets worse on lying on the back and during the night.
- IPECAC: When accompanied with nausea, vomiting, a rattling sound in the throat and lungs 3X or 6 will do.
- BRYONIA: When there is dry cough with stitching pain in the chest, difficult expectoration which gets worse on going to a warm place from a cold one.
- BELLADONNA: For whooping cough of children. The face becomes red while coughing, cough due to throat trouble, worse at night.
- CALCAREA CARB.: When there is cough after the first sleep, thin, sweet expectoration, expectoration is pus like and if put in a cup of water it sinks to the bottom.

- ANTIM TART.: When there is difficult breathing, the patient cannot expectorate, and his hands and feet are cold.
- SULPHUR: For chronic cough.
- DROSERA: For whooping cough, which gets worse on laughing, weeping, singing, or smoking, and the face becomes red on coughing.
- MAGNESIA PHOS.: Spasmodic cough is relieved by giving it dissolved in hot water, 3X or 6X.
- SPONGIA: For dry, barking cough, which has a whistling sound.
- HEPAR: For very old cough which gets worse during cold.
- PULSATILLA: When there is yellow expectoration, and coughing gets better in open air.
- PHOSPHORUS: When there is salty, rusty, expectoration, and the cough is excited when the patient goes to a cool place from a warm one. 30 or 200 once a day or a week.
- NUX VOM.: When the cough is due to indigestion.
- KALI BICHROM: When there is stingy and ropy expectoration which gets worse after meals or about 3 a.m
- KALI CARB.: When it gets worse about 4 a.m.
- GRAPHITES: When there is whooping cough and the patient passes urine or stool with cough.
- COCCUS CACTI: When it gets worse in winter but is better on drinking cold water or in a cool place, and worse in a warm room or on taking a warm drink.
- BROMIUM: When it occurs during summer due to dust. One dose in 2-3 days.

TUBERCULOSIS

This is a serious disease, but the discovery of antibiotics has made it curable. The Bacillus Tuberculosis enters the body with the breath and attacks the lungs, deteriorating them. Fever, cough, debility are common symptoms. The patient loses weight. The bacilli can be detected in the sputum of the patient by microscopic examination. Those who are weak in health can contact the disease from any T.B. patient but those who are healthy will not. Open air is essential for a T.B. patient. Living conditions in cities are responsible for this disease. Anxiety, disappointment, loss in business, grief, mortification, humiliation etc. are also some of the causes of T.B.

Antibiotics like Streptomycin, Pas, Isonex do arrest the disease but even after that the patient should live in healthy surroundings, otherwise a relapse may occur.

The Christian missionaries of the Methodist church did successfully treat many cases of T.B. by Naturopathic methods. Mud plasters, breathing exercises, open air resorts, breathing from a wet pit, etc. are some of the methods they used. Homoeopathic medicines have cured many cases which were treated in early stages. A few medicines are given below.

- TUBERCULINUM and BACILLINUM: These medicines are prepared from tubercular lungs. Patients from a hot climate will respond to TUBERCULINUM and those from damp places will be benefited by the BACILLINUM. Never use less than 30 potency, 200 or 1000 is better. These should not be repeated before a week or month. Slight but constant fever, with cold catarrh, cough, etc. are the primary symptoms when these medicines will avert the attack.
- ARSENIC IODIDE 3X TRIT.: This remedy is said to be the head remedy for T.B. This may be given when there is an evening rise of temperature and the pulse proportionately rapid. Normally the pulse rate is 72, when the temperature is normal (98.4 degrees). With the rise of one degree in temperature the pulse will heat 10-12 times more; but if the beats are more than 10-12 times per degree, T.B. should be suspected and ARSENIC IODIDE 3X should be given 2-3 times daily, dry on the tongue

after meals. Liquid drinks should be avoided for about 1 hour. The phial of ARSENIC IODIDE 3X should be kept in a dark place covered with dark paper. Light decomposes it. Reputed Homoeopathic physicians of U.S.A. have recommended 21 medicines for T.B. They are:

1. IODIUM
2. CALCAREA IODIDE 3X TRIT.
3. MERC PROTO IODIDE 3X TRIT.
4. ARS. IODIDE 3X TRIT.
5. PHOS. 30, 200
6. CALCAREA PHOS. 12X TRIT.
7. TUBERCULINUM 200, 1000
8. FERRUM MET. 30
9. CALCAREA CARB. 3
10. PULS 3, 30
11. THYRO. 30
12. SULPHUR 30, 200
13. HYDRASTIS
14. NUX MOSCHATA
15. GALIC ACID
16. ACID PHOS.
17. ACID MUR.
18. ERYNGIUM
19. IPECAC
20. GERANIUM and
21. ACID NIT.

In addition to these remedies which should be studied in the *Materia Medica,* we have also found the following medicines quite useful:

- BAPTISIA 1X, FERRUM PHOS. 6X, ACONITE 3X, ECHINACEA Q, PYROGENIUM 30 in fever.
- JABORANDI for profuse sweats.

- GENTIANA Q for loss of appetite.
- ACALYPHA INDICA, GERANIUM and IPECAC for bleeding.

The climate of hill stations is very conducive in this disease; open air is a must. A nutritious diet and freedom from worry and anxiety are also needed.

13

HEART DISEASES

The heart is the most important organ in the human body. Its structure is very delicate. The ailments of the heart are very complicated and serious. Therefore, when a heart disease is suspected, senior physicians should be consulted. Here we are mentioning remedies of some common diseases of the heart. If given in the beginning they will arrest the diseases and give relief to the patient.

PALPITATION

Ordinarily our heart beats 72 times in a minute and these beats are responsible for the circulation of blood in the whole body. When there is some disease of the heart these beats are increased in number. This is called palpitation. The beats are increased even without disease of the heart, for example, when there is anaemia (poor blood), anxiety, grief, loss of vital fluids, over-indulgence, fear, shame, mortification, or drinking. During palpitation the patient is restless and anxious. To cure him the cause should be removed.

- CACTUS Q: 4-5 drops in an ounce of water should be taken twice or thrice daily.

- IBERIS Q: When there is pain in the region of the heart, palpitation is worse on coughing or any other kind of exertion, the patient has constriction in the throat and vertigo.
- ACONITE 1X or 3X: The patient feels as if his heart will stop suddenly; there is fear of death. Patient is anguished and restless.
- NATRUM MUR.: When there is missing of pulse or palpitation due to emotional causes grief, disappointment, worry etc., a dose of 200 will do.
- ARNICA: When it is due to injury, accident, etc.
- CACTUS Q or 30: When the patient has the feeling as if his heart was being squeezed with an iron band.
- CHINA: When there is extreme debility due to a loss of vital fluids.
- LACHESIS, DIGITALIS and SPIGELIA should also be studied.

HEART ATTACK (ANGINA PECTORIS)

The pain is not due to any defect in the heart itself but it is due to some defect either in the muscles or nerves of the heart. Smoking, drinking, worries or rheumatism are also its causes. A shooting pain starts suddenly in the left chest and travels up to the left shoulder and arm. Dyspnoea, restlessness, rapid breathing and cold sweats occur and sometimes the patient becomes unconscious. At the time of pain often a few drops of Amyl nitrite are put on a handkerchief and placed at the nose of the patient. It gives relief.

During the attack the pain is severe, rather unbearable. Take half a cup of hot water and dissolve 5 tablets each of MAGNESIA PHOS. 6X and KALI PHOS. 6X and administer spoonful doses every 5 minutes. This will relieve the pain. In case there is fear of death, extreme restlessness and anguish, ACONITE 1X or 3X drop doses should be given every 15 minutes.

- ARSENIC A.: When there is extreme restlessness, great debility, unquenchable thirst and burning, and the patient feels that he is dying. Give 30, 200 every half hour or 2 hours.
- DIGITALIS Q or 30: When there is a feeling that the heart was gradually sinking.
- AURUM: When there is rapid pulse and the feeling as if the heart beats stopped for 2-3 seconds.
- CACTUS 1X, 30: When there is pain extending to the left shoulder and arm and feeling of iron band on the heart.
- SPIGELIA: When the patient cannot lie on the left side and is worse at the least motion. Sometimes the pain extends to hands and legs, and he feels better on taking a hot drink or lying on the right side.
- CRATAEGUS Q: This is a tonic for the heart. 5-10 drops twice daily will avert the attacks; it should be continued for some time.
- ACID HYDRO.: When there are frequent attacks.

Sometimes the attacks are due to some defect in the heart itself or its blood vessels. Then the above mentioned medicines are useful, specially SPIGELIA and SPONGIA.

BLOOD PRESSURE

Nowadays there is much unnecessary propaganda of Blood Pressure. If any one feels a little headache he goes to his physician and asks him to check his blood pressure. Doctors too when they examine the patient, will check his blood pressure without fail, and will express anxiety about it, but the fact is that Blood Pressure is not a disease in itself but only a symptom of a disease. When our blood vessels — veins and arteries — become a bit stiff due to old age or disease of the heart, liver or kidney, the pressure in the blood vessels increases. Normally when the heart contracts the blood pressure is between 130-160, and 90-120 when it dilates. It is less when one is younger and high in old age. It is normally believed that one's age plus 100 is his normal B.P.

Dull headache, heaviness of head even without pain, loss of sleep, dyspnoea, anguish and restlessness are some symptoms of B.P. It becomes normal after a disease of the heart, liver or kidneys is treated successfully. Sometimes it rises due to anxiety, worry, loss in business, disappointment in love or due to failure in examination or defeat in elections etc. This rise is temporary and time cures it.

IGNATIA and ACID PHOS. are its head remedies. Mahatma Gandhi had B.P. but he took no medicines to keep it down. He used to take garlic and kept cold mud plaster on his head when there was a rise in his B.P.

Rest, reduction in the quantity of food, more drinking of water and keeping oneself free from worries are necessary to keep one's B.P. normal.

- BARYTA CARB. 6, 30 TRIT.: The chief remedy of High Blood Pressure, specially for persons over 50.
- BARYTA MUR. 3X TRIT.: When the difference between the systolic and diastolic pressure is abnormal, i.e., more than 40-50, 3-4 grains be given dry on tongue twice daily.
- CONIUM: When there is vertigo from least motion of head, aversion to exertion, trembling of legs and palpitation of heart. Suits old maids.
- BELLADONNA 3X or 30: In acute cases repeat every half hour. Headache will be relieved and the patient will sleep.
- GLONOINE 6, 30: When it is worse in summer and sun, there is pain in temples, the patient feels his head has become bigger.
- SANGUINARIA: When the cheeks are red and the patient gets worse in light and better in a dark room; headache increases with sunrise and decreases after sunset.

- GELS.: When the tongue is dry and it trembles.
- LACHESIS, IGNATIA, NATRUM MUR. and AURUM MET. are some other medicines which are indicated in High Blood Pressure.

LOW BLOOD PRESSURE

In some disease the blood pressure falls below normal which is not good. Sometimes it falls due to worry and anxiety or in some debilitating diseases.

- CACTUS Q: A few drops with water will normalise L.B.P. Give hourly or two hourly.
- CRATAEGUS Q: 5-10 drops twice or thrice daily will keep it normal.
- LYCOPODIUM: If L.B.P. is worse and occurs between 4-8 p.m.
- NATRUM MUR.: When it is due to mental or emotional causes.
- CHINA: When it is due to a loss of vital fluids.
- SEPIA and CARBO VEG. should also be considered.

There are several other heart diseases but their diagnosis and treatment should be left to professional physicians.

14

MENTAL DISORDERS

We shall now deal with diseases which attack the head which contains the most important organ of human body, the brain. It is the centre from where nerves go to every part of our body. The brain controls all our bodily functions through this nervous system. A defect or any irregularity in the brain will result in mental and bodily ailments. Homoeopathy has a good reputation in the treatment of mental diseases. Here is a brief account of the mental derailments and their treatment.

EPILEPSY

In this disease a patient suddenly falls down and becomes unconscious. He has violent breathing, froths from the mouth, and has convulsions and cramps in the whole body.

- OENANTHE CROCATA Q: When there are attacks during menses or due to suppressed menses. Sometimes the patient vomits. Mother tincture, one or two drops 2-3 times daily.
- ARTEMISIA Q: When the disease is due to worms or during dentition or due to injury to heat or due to some grief,

fear or mortification. Two drops in water or fruit juice 3-4 times daily will avert repeated attacks.

- IGNATIA: When the disease is due to humiliation, grief, fear, disappointment or loss.
- CAUSTICUM: Tension in chest and abdomen precedes attack; during attack the head is drawn on one side. Involuntary urination. Headache and debility after the attack. Often the tongue is bitten. Attacks occur about new moon. If the disease is due to the suppression of eczema or any skin disease, CAUSTICUM will cure it.
- CUPRUM MET.: Often the attack is sudden, with a shriek and falling down, without any premonitory signs. During attack involuntary discharge of urine, chest and head covered with perspiration. After the attack weeping, trembling, shaking of right hand and sleep.

Homoeopathy has cured many incurable epilepsy patients but the selection of the correct medicine is rather difficult. Here we are giving names of a few medicines with their important symptoms. For details, *Materia Medica* may be consulted.

- SILICEA: Attacks mostly occur during sleep. There are records of three patients who had attacks while sleeping only, during the day or night. SILICEA 200, 1000 and CM at long intervals cured the patients and they never had an attack for the last 10-12 years.
- CALCAREA CARB.: Suits fat persons, attacks about full moon.
- BUFO, LACHESIS and DIGITALIS: For persons who have practised masturbation and are sexually weak. 200 or 1000 potency should be used.
- ARGENTUM NIT.: Epilepsy due to over smoking. 200 potency every week.
- SEPIA: When the attack occurs once in a week or once in two or three weeks. Time of attacks is mostly morning. Head turns to the left.

- SULPHUR, TARENTULA, CICUTA, HYOSCYAMUS and ARSENIC: May be used according to symptoms. We had a patient who was prescribed CUPRUM according to symptoms. There was partial relief in the intensity of attacks but the attacks recurred every 31st day. There are two medicines in Homoeopathy which have periodicity: ARSENIC and CHINA. ARSENIC was tried but in vain. Then CHINA 1000 was given and after a week CUPRUM 1000. For the last 4-5 years the patient did not have any attack. Now he takes CHINA 1000 once a month and CUPRUM 1000 once in three months.

INSANITY, MANIA OR MADNESS

There are many different kinds of this disease and a mad man exhibits different symptoms at different times. Sometimes he is dumb, sometimes talkative, sometimes he escapes from home or is violent and bites, tears clothes, swears, weeps, laughs, sings, handles organs or has delusions of various kinds. You will find here a few medicines with their chief symptoms. Homoeopathy gives great importance to mental symptoms and many incurable cases of mental diseases have been completely cured by properly selected drugs.

- STRAMONIUM: Excited state, patient thinks his whole body or a part or organ has increased in size, becomes very irritable, bites, abuses, talks foolishly, laughs, acts, feels restless, desires to go away, has visions of ghosts, fights with them, has visions of animals, is excited sexually, wants to be kissed, talks lewdly, does not like to remain alone, fears darkness, wants light, has fits on looking at water or a glaring, shining thing, prays, weeps laughs, gives religious sermons, fears death.
- BELLADONNA: Severe headache, dilated pupils, the patient has illusions of senses, beautiful or frightful images of

ghosts, insects, bats, black dogs that will bite, devils, soldiers and executioners who want to take away the patient, growling and barking like dogs, singing, whistling, dancing. Becomes violent, strikes, bites.

- HYOSCYAMUS: The patient is shameless, becomes naked, has sexual mania, prays to gods, laughs, sings. Handles private organs, is jealous and suspicious, fears that he will be poisoned, repeats a thing again and again.
- IGNATIA: For insanity or mental symptoms caused by grief, anxiety, fear, sorrow, disappointment, or mortification. Silent brooding, singing; the patient thinks he or she has committed some crime; symptoms caused by loss of dear ones or dear things or by loss in business. If a child has been scolded or punished and mental symptoms appear after that, this is the chief remedy; alternative and contradictory symptoms such as cries and laughs, or is happy and then very sad.
- SULPHUR: The patient regards rags as beautiful clothes and decorates himself with them; likes and wears rags of different colours. Is dirty, does not like to be washed; is selfish, uncharitable, irritable, quarrelsome, short tempered: aggravation before the new moon and at 11 a.m.; anxious about the salvation of his soul, proud. Disgusting smell from the body. Good for old cases.
- ACONITE: The patient fears death, predicts the day of his death; feels anxious and restless; fear of crowds and crossing the street. Sticks to one thought.
- ANACARDIUM: The patient has impaired memory, swears again and again, is irritable and suspicious, timid and apprehensive. Thinks he is surrounded by enemies, hears voices of dead persons or of those who are far off. Sees a bier in the next room upon which he himself or a friend is lying as corpse; thinks as he is possessed of two person or wills, out of which one tells him to do a certain thing and the other prevents. Thinks he is being pursued.

Profound melancholy and hypochondriasis, with a tendency to use violent language absent-minded, very easily offended. Malicious, seems bent upon wickedness, has lack of confidence in himself and others. Suspicious, absence of all moral restraints.

- AGARICUS: Makes poems, sings, talks but does not answer. Talkative but indifferent, has aversion to work, make prophecies. Fearless, wants to hurt others.
- AMMONIUM CARB.: The patient is sad, weeps, is unreasonable. Forgetful, ill humoured, gloomy during stormy weather. Thinks he is sinful, is weary of life, flatulence, fears water, does not want to be washed, aggravation during menses.
- AMMONIUM MUR.: Insanity caused by grief or sorrow. The patient wants to cry but cannot, there is offensive sweat in the soles. He feels icy coldness between both the shoulders, and is better in open air.
- APIS MEL.: The patient is awkward, drops things easily, is jealous, fidgety, wants to run or jump, has fear of death. Insanity of the widows due to suppression of sex.
- ARGENTUM NIT.: The patient wants to jump out of the window, fixes the day of his death, is hasty, nervous, melancholic, impulsive.
- ARNICA: Insanity due to head injury. Head feels hot, body is cold. The patient fears to be touched, wants to be left alone, has fear of space. He is nervous, morose, after a mental shock or strain.
- ARSENIC ALB.: The patient has fear of death, extreme prostration, is afraid of ghosts and thieves. Has fear of lice, wants to hide himself and to live alone. Is devoid of hope, anxious, anguished and considers himself worthless and sinful. Has hallucinations of smell and sight. Is miserly, malicious, selfish, lacks courage, and is sensitive especially to disorder and confusion.
- AURUM MET.: The patient has a tendency to suicide but fears death. Is hasty, disgusted with life, has a feeling of

self-condemnation and utter worthlessness. There is profound despondency with increased blood pressure and constant rapid questioning without waiting for reply.

- CALCAREA CARB.: Insanity of drunkards, insanity due to suppression of skin disease. Dementia. The patient is apprehensive, fears loss of reason, misfortune or a contagious disease. Is forgetful, confused, low spirited, has aversion to work.
- CALCAREA PHOS.: Insanity of young men, specially due to masturbation or sexual excesses or due to grief and anger. The patient wants to wander and thinks of going somewhere, while living at home.
- CANNABIS INDICA: The patient has uncontrollable laughter, time passes slowly, seconds seem like ages, a few yards an immense distance. He has fear of being insane, is talkative yet very forgetful; while talking forgets what is to be said further. He discusses principles, has hallucinations, sees imaginary things.
- CAUSTICUM: Insanity due to excessive anxiety, grief, sorrow, quarrel, etc. The patient always thinks about and sees the dark side of everything. Feels as if the portion between the skull and brain is empty. Cannot see others in trouble. Disease due to suppression of skin disease.
- CICUTA: Disease due to suppression of eruptions. Indifference to surroundings, the patient feels as if things are strange and fearful; keeps singing, dancing, clapping. Has confidence in no one.
- CIMICIFUGA: Insanity due to repeated losses in business or failure in undertakings, or due to suppression of neuralgic pains. The patient feels as if he has been covered from all sides; dreams of imaginary evils, suspects everybody, does not even take medicine from others. Talks much and changes topics one after the other. Feels as if rats were roaming around him. Has a suicidal

tendency, fear of death, disappointment in love. Wants to walk alone.

- COCCULUS: Mania due to excessive sexual indulgence or constant night watching. The patient is very sad, anxious, feels that time is passing quickly. He cannot remain without singing, cannot bear contradiction. Has anxiety about the health of others.
- CROCUS SATIVA: The patient keeps singing and laughing, is joyful, kisses everybody yet suddenly becomes angry, quick changes in moods.
- KALI BROM.: The patient apprehends that someone may poison him. Is always busy with shoes, typing and loosening them. Feels his pockets. Picks straws. Thinks there is a conspiracy against him. Has night terrors. Imagines he is singled out as an object of divine wrath.
- KALI PHOS.: Disease due to overwork. Nervous dread. The patient does not want to mix up with people. Slightest labour seems a heavy task.
- LACHESIS: The patient is very talkative, has no desire to mix with people. Has a religious mania, delusions, regards day as night and night as day. Ill effects of suppressed discharges. Derangement of time sense, feels suspicious. Mental labour, best performed at night.
- LYCOPODIUM: The patient is sad, has a lack of self-confidence. He is apprehensive, thinks he is ill and feels that he is at two places at the same time. Weeps and laughs alternately, cannot collect his thoughts.
- NATRUM MUR.: Psychic causes of disease, ill effects of grief, fright, anger, etc. The patient resents consoling. He is irritable, wants to be alone to cry. Has tears with laughter, is depressed.
- MEDORRHINUM: Time passes too slowly. The patient is afraid of going insane. Cannot speak without weeping. Melancholy with suicidal thoughts.
- NUX VOMICA: The patient is fidgety, cannot bear noise and light. Is irritable, angry, does not want to be touched.

Time passes too slowly. He is disposed to reproach others, sullen, fault finding.

- PHOSPHORUS: The patient has sexual mania, thinks that he is a very important person. Has fear of death when alone. Restless, fidgety.
- PLATINA: The patient feels proud, has contempt of others. There is self exaltation. Has an irresistible impulse to kill. Mental troubles associated with suppressed menses. Physical symptoms disappear as mental symptoms develop.
- PULSATILLA: The patient weeps easily, feels timid, irresolute, likes sympathy. Has a religion mania, prays for his and others' salvation. Fears opposite sex. Thinks his action are unpardonable. Is afraid of ghosts at night when alone.
- RHUS TOX.: The patient has fear of being poisoned, has a suicidal tendency by drowning, extreme restlessness, sadness.
- SILICEA: The patient thinks that a hair is sticking to his tongue, clears it again and again. Imagines of pins, collects them, counts them.
- TARENTULA HISPANICA: The patient sings, dances, laughs, pricks, cuts jokes, picks hair. Throws or destroys whatever he gets. He is foxy, has a stealing tendency. Does not like others to sing or dance.
- ZINCUM MET.: Melancholia. The patient repeats everything that is said to him. Disease after suppression of skin diseases. Fears he will be arrested. Dislikes noise.
- THUJA: The patient thinks he is made of glass. Music makes him tremble and weep. Does not want to be touched or looked at. Has fixed ideas as if a strange person was at his side, as if his soul and body were separated, as if there was something alive in his abdomen.
- VERATRUM ALBUM: Mania with a desire to cut and tear things. The patient sits in a stupid manner, notices

nothing. Strikes, curses. Has delusions of impending misfortune.

- ALUMINA: The patient is hasty, has a suicidal tendency by cutting his throat but fears death. Alternate moods.
- ARGENTUM MET.: The patient is hasty. Time passes slowly. He is melancholy, restless, feels as if his body is being dilated.
- BARYTA CARB.: The patient is shy, does not want to meet unknown persons. Childish behaviour.
- LILIUM TIG.: The patient fears he has some organic and incurable disease. He feels aimless, hurried. He curses, strikes, thinks of obscene matters. Profound depression of spirits. Consolation aggravates it. Is hasty.
- VERATRUM VIR.: Insanity due to high blood pressure or rush of blood to the head. The patient is silent, does not talk even with the physician.
- STAPHISAGRIA: Disease caused by shock to one's self respect, or as a result of insult, anger, etc. The patient is sad, hypochondriacal. Sensitive to what others say about him.
- SPIGELIA: The patient is afraid of sharp pointed things, pins, needles, spears, etc.
- SEPIA: The patient is sad, morose, irritable, easily offended. Dreads to be alone. Indifferent to loved ones. Miserly, weeps when telling symptoms.
- CROTALUS: The patient hates his own family members. Wants to escape and hide himself. Talks much, is impatient.
- CONIUM: Disease due to suppression of sexual desires. The patient wants to be alone, feels depressed, timid, takes no interest in anything. Memory gets weak.
- CHAMOMILLA: The patient wants to be praised by others. Feels insulted on trifles.
- ABSINTHIUM: The patient has kleptomania, is brutal. Forgets what recently happened. Keeps talking on any one subject repeatedly.

- COFFEA: The patient feels remorse, and is repentant, very sad.

There is such a wide variety in mental diseases that the above-mentioned drugs may not be sufficient. Yet more drugs may be studied and tried. Mental symptoms of all the drugs have been carefully marked and noted in Homoeopathy.

15

URINARY PROBLEMS

CALCULUS (STONE)

Stone is found either in kidneys or in bladder. When this stone moves from kidneys towards bladder through ureter there is agonising pain. After the stone passes out the pain is relieved. Hot fomentation on the back as well as lower abdomen is always useful.

- BERBERIS V. Q: During pain 5 drops in an ounce of hot water should be repeated every 15-20 minutes.
- MAGNESIA PHOS 3X: 5 grains or 5 tablets dissolved in hot water and given repeatedly relieves the pain.
- STIGMATA MAYDIS Q: 15-20 drops in hot water during pain relieves it.
- SARSAPARILLA 30, DIOSCOREA Q, PAREIRA BRAVA Q and THLASPI BURSA PASTORIS Q are also very useful.

When the pain is relieved the following medicines should be given to prevent recurrence of pain and expel the stone.

- LYCO.: When there is a reddish sediment in urine.

- URTICA URENS Q: 5 drops in water 2-3 times a day. Continue for some days.
- ACID PHOS. 3X: When phosphates are found in urine.
- GRAPHITES: When the sediment in urine smells sour.
- CHIN SULPH. 3X: When the sediment in urine is reddish or brownish in colour.
- LITHIUM CARB. 3X TRIT.: When the stone is in bladder, continue twice daily for some days. It dissolves and expels the bladder stone.
- SARSAPARILLA, OXALIC ACID and NITRO MURIATIC ACID should also be studied.

INFLAMMATION IN KIDNEYS (NEPHRITIS)

Is a pretty serious disease. Pain, fever, restlessness, dyspnoea are its usual symptoms. As the kidneys being involved do not function, the toxins or poisons which are not excreted mix with the blood resulting in uraemia, unconsciousness and even collapse. Such cases should be entrusted to experienced physicians. A few medicines are given below.

- ACONITE 3X: To be given in the beginning, during fever, restlessness, etc.
- TEREBINTHINA: When the quantity of urine decreases.
- CAMPHOR Q: On sudden retention of urine. In babies it may be smelt by putting the phial near the nose of the baby.
- NUX., IGNATIA, GELS., PULS. etc. are also indicated.

INFLAMMATION OF URINARY BLADDER (CYSTITIS)

The symptoms generally begin with retention of urine, pain on passing urine, dribbling chill and fever.

- CANTHARIS 3X, 30: Chief remedy when it occurs with burning.

- DULCAMARA: If the cause is dampness, getting wet in rain.
- ACONITE 3X: When due to dry cold winds.
- CHAMOMILLA: In chronic cases.
- PAREIRA BRAVA Q: 2-3 drops 2-5 times daily when kidney is also involved.
- ACID BENZOIC: If there is offensive odour in urine, just like a horse's urine.
- ACID NITRIC: When there is repulsive bad odour.
- BELLADONNA, CAUSTICUM, PULS., CANN. SATIVA and SABAL SERRULATA Q should also be consulted.

DIABETES

When sugar is found in urine, it is termed diabetes. Patient becomes weaker and weaker, losses flesh, is emaciated. One Major O'Mera, Inspector General of Hospitals, in his book on tropical diseases says that he cured many diabetic patients by keeping them on Dab (watery juice in fresh coconut) for 2-3 months. Walking is said to be the best treatment for diabetes. I have known many cases who lived long up to the age of 80-85 though they contacted diabetes in middle age, by taking recourse to walking for 8 to 12 miles daily, preferably in early morning hours. Lemon, papaya, *bel*, *mooli* (radish), *bengan* (brinjal), *karela* and *jamun* are said to be efficacious in controlling diabetes.

- SYZYGIUM JAMBOLANUM Q: Most useful; no other remedy causes in so marked a degree the diminution and disappearance of sugar in urine.
- NATRUM SULPH. 6X and NATRUM PHOS. 6X: Specific remedies for diabetes. Both should be taken one in morning and the other in the night continuously for some days.
- LACTIC ACID: When there is pain in joint also.
- SECALE COR.: When there is much thirst, burning in palms and soles.
- PLUMBUM IODIDE: When uric acid increases.

- ARGENTUM MET.: When there is swelling on feet.
- TEREBINTHINA: When there is burning in urine, albumin also passes with sugar.

Other Medicines: ACID PHOS., CEPHALANDRA, HELONIAS, RHUS and NATRUM MUR.

INVOLUNTARY PASSING OF URINE (ENURESIS)

The disease is found mostly in children, but adults also are sometime found suffering from it.

- FERRUM PHOS 12x, 200x: To be given twice daily for some time in 12x. 200x should be repeated twice a week only.
- BELLADONNA: If the patient wets the bed during sleep.
- CAUSTICUM: When the patient passes urine before midnight.
- SEPIA: When there is offensive urine.
- CANTHARIS: When the patient passes urine while sleeping. during the day.
- CINA: When the patient has a history of worms.
- NATRUM PHOS.: When it is due to worms.
- SULPHUR: In chronic cases.

16

MALE SEX DISEASES

IMPOTENCE

Inability in a man to achieve an erection or orgasm.

- NUPHAR LUTEUM Q: When there is a complete absence of erections, pain in testicles, parts relaxed. Two drops two times daily for some time.
- LYCOPODIUM: For impotency in old age.
- SABAL SERRULATA Q: When the testicles are shrunk, penis cold, 5-10 drops twice or thrice daily.
- ONOSMODIUM: When there is incomplete erection, too speedy emission.
- CALADIUM: For impotency due to masturbation, violent desire but penis is loose.
- STAPHYSAGRIA: When it is due to excess.

INCREASED DESIRE

- PHOSPHORUS: When there are frequent erections, uncontrollable sexual thoughts. Suits young persons.

- CONIUM: When due to bad effects of suppressed desire, emission on slightest emotion.
- ORIGANUM: When someone takes to masturbation due to excessive desire.
- TARENTULA H.: When there is great excitement.

MASTURBATION

- BUFO: When the person seeks solitude to practise masturbation.
- USTILAGO Q: When there is an irresistible tendency to masturbation, the person is despondent, has sexual dreams.
- CONIUM: For bad effects of masturbation.
- CALADIUM: Like USTILAGO it controls the habit and removes its bad effects.
- ORIGANUM: When the person is mad after the practise.
- HYOSCYAMUS: When the person is shameless, plays with organs, has uncontrollable desire for masturbation.

SEMINAL EMISSIONS (SPERMATORRHOEA)

A nocturnal emission is a spontaneous orgasm during sleep that includes ejaculation for a male. Nocturnal emissions are most common during adolescence and early young adult years, but they may happen any time after puberty.

- SELENIUM: Chief remedy. When there is emission with urine, at the time of passing stools, during coition emission is too rapid with long lasting thrill.
- SULPHUR: When there is emission before the erection is complete.
- BARYTA CARB.: When there are emissions in night-dreams, desire is diminished.

- THUJA Q: 5 drops twice daily is very useful for emissions whether during dreams or otherwise
- BELLIS PERENNIS Q: 5 drops twice daily for all sorts of emissions.
- GELSEMIUM: When there is emission without dream.
- AGNUS CASTUS: In acute cases of impotency. Desire much but no erection, cold organs. In chronic cases when even the desire is lost.
- PHOS. ACID: When there are night-dreams, loss of memory, sudden relaxation before emission.
- CHINA: For debility due to emissions. When there is singing in ears, vertigo.
- PHOSPHORUS: When there is early emission during coition, palpitation, organ is relaxed.
- PICRIC ACID: When the person has terrible erections and great desire.
- GRAPHITES: When there is absence of emission.
- SEPIA: When there is insufficient erection.
- STAPHISAGRIA: For bad effects of masturbation, when there are dark rings about the eyes, a sallow face, the person is why and peevish.
- LYCO.: When there is complete impotency, erections absent, emission frequent.
- DIOSCOREA: When there are two or three dreams in the night with emissions, the person has weakness about the knees.
- ERYNGIUM AQUATICUM 2X: Very efficacious for emissions with or without erections.

PENIS PROBLEMS

- COCA and COCAINE: When there are sensations as if the penis was absent.
- KREOSOTE: When there is burning during coition, swelling.

- CAUSTICUM: When there is itching on penis.
- IGNATIA: When the penis is small and retracted.
- NUPHAR: For retraction.
- LYCO.: When the penis becomes small due to masturbation.
- PHIMOSIS: When the foreskin sticks to penis, cannot be drawn over.
- NITRIC ACID: When the penis has swelling.

Prostate: There are two glands at the root of penis, when they are enlarged or inflamed and cause urinary troubles.

- BARYTA CARB.: When there is enlargement in old age, frequent urination.
- ARNICA: When there is enlargement or swelling due to injury.
- THUJA: When the penis is effected due to gonorrhoea.
- SABAL SERRULATA Q: 10 drops twice daily often avoids operation.
- PAREIRA: With retention of urine.
- FERRUM PICRICUM 3X TRIT.: Twice or thrice daily reduces enlargement.
- TRITICUM REPENS Q or 30: When the bladder is irritable.
- PULSATILLA: In acute cases, with pain in testicles.
- MERC. SOL.: When there is a tendency to suppuration or pus has formed.
- CHIMAPHILA Q: 3-4 drops twice daily has often cured.
- CONIUM, STAPHYSAGRIA, IODIUM, SOLIDAGO and OCIMUM CANUM should also be studied.

ORCHITIS

Inflammation and swelling of testicles.

- ACONITE: When it is accompanied with fever.
- PULS.: In acute cases.

- BELL.: For red swelling.
- HAMAMELIS: When there is much swelling and tension.
- APIS: When there is stinging pain, swelling but not deep, only in outer covering. Oedematous whitish swelling.
- SPONGIA, ARNICA, AURUM, MERC. SOL. and CLEMATIS may also be studied.

HYDROCELE

Collection of fluid in scrotum, the sac of testicles.

- SPONGIA: When it occurs with throbbing pain.
- RHODODENDRON: When the right side is effected, gets worse during stormy weather.
- PULS.: For left sided hydrocele.
- APIS: When there is shining oedematous swelling.

GONORRHOEA

This disease is contacted by coition with a person of other sex. In the beginning there is burning and pus in urine. When the poison spreads there is pain in joints, inflammation of eyes and warts. Antibiotics, like penicillin, it is claimed neutralise the poison.

- CANNABIS INDICA Q: When the patient has reached an acute stage, there is terrible burning in urine which extends to bladder. Thick yellowish pus, tension in testicles, phimosis, urine in drops.
- CANTHARIS: When there is frequent but scanty urine, pus with blood.
- PETROSELINUM Q: 5-6 drops twice or thrice daily relieves the agonising pain in urination and reduces pus, etc.
- THUJA: To cure the aftereffects of the disease, warts, pain in joints, gout. Use 200-1000 potency infrequently.
- OLEUM SANTALI Q: When there is swelling in glans, thick yellowish pus.

- NATRUM SULPH.: For chilly patients, in chronic cases.
- COPAIVA Q: When there is a milky white discharge. Suited to women.
- SEPIA: For ladies.
- MEDORRHINUM 200: In chronic cases. When the patient has rheumatism and gout.
- KALI SULPH. 6X: In chronic cases. When there is greenish discharge.
- MERC. COR.: When the foreskin sticks, cannot remove either side, thick greenish discharge red orifice swollen.
- GELS.: When there is much pain, soreness.
- HYDRASTIS Q: When there is a thick yellow discharge, urine offensive, pus.
- ACONITE: To be given in the beginning, when there is fever.
- NITRIC ACID: When it occurs owing to an abuse of mercury.

SYPHILIS

This disease is also contacted after coition with a person of opposite sex suffering from syphilis. There occur buboes near testicles, ulcers on genitals. This disease was brought to India by the English people, it is therefore, popularly known as *Phirang Rog*.

- MERC. SOL.: Chief remedy. It should be given as soon as eruption is seen on penis.
- MERC. PROTO IODIDE: It follows MERC. SOL. and continuous use of 3x or 6x for some days often cures the disease.
- KALI IODIDE: In lower potencies for some days gives relief.
- SYPHILINUM: 200, 1000 weekly or monthly cures old cases.
- NITRIC ACID: If the malady occurs after abuse of mercury.
- PHYTOLACCA: When there are buboes at the root of the thighs.
- SILICEA: When there is pus in ulcers.

- AURUM MET.: When there are ulcers in the eyes or nose.
- MEZEREUM: When there is pain in bones.
- THUJA, HEPAR, ARS, CINNABARIS, KALI IOD. and GRAPHITES are also found useful.

17

SOME MORE DISEASES

CANCER

Although there is no cure for cancer yet, detecting and treating the disease at an early stage can significantly improve a person's outlook.

Cancer is a disease that causes cells to grow and multiply uncontrollably in certain parts of the body. In the beginning it appears in the form of a small tumor without pain. If it persists for a month or so, Homoeopathic treatment should be started. If treatment is started early 75 percent of the cases are likely to be cured.

The tumor may appear on the tongue, cheek or any place on the outer body, inside the nose, throat, in the uterus of women, breasts, in the stomach, lungs, liver, etc. If this tumor is cancerous it gradually increases in size and destroys the tissues. An abcess is formed which ultimately turns into an ulcer or even gangrene. To ascertain whether the tumor is cancerous, a small piece of it is examined which is termed as Biopsy. If the result is positive no treatment is possible. If the tumor is removed by operation the cancer appears elsewhere. Sometimes the poison attacks the blood which is termed as Lukemia or Blood Cancer.

Some scientists are of the opinion that mental tension due to disappointment in love, loss in business or any kind of grief, sorrow, mortification results in cancer. Smoking or chewing of tobacco is responsible for more than 30 percent cases of cancer.

The following medicines have been found useful in this disease.

- CARCINOSIN: 200 or 1000 can be given in all kinds of cases inter currently with other indicated medicines weekly or monthly.
- CONIUM: 200 or 1000 have cured many cases. It is specially useful for cancer of the breasts or places where there are thick muscles.
- ARS.: When burning predominates.
- KALI CYANATUM 30, 200: It has cured tongue cancers specially in cases where the patient had neuralgia of face.
- HYDRASTIS Q: Useful specially in the cancer of uterus. Its lotion should be used for douching the parts. It allays pain. 200 potency should be given weekly.
- CARBO ANIMALIS 3X, 30: When it bursts and pus comes out.
- ACONITE RADIX: For relieving pains give one or two drops in an ounce of water every one or two hours until the pain is relieved.
- RADIUM BROM 30. and SELENIUM 30: In all cases once a week.
- PHOS. 30, 200: In cancer of mouth, throat, lips or cheek. The patient craves ice cold water because ice relieves pain. Many patients have been benefited by it.
- PHOS.: It has also cured cancer of the stomach when in addition to the above symptoms the patient vomits water as soon as it gets warm in the stomach.
- HEKLA LAVA 3X TRIT.: For cancer of bones.
- CONDURANGO: Its guiding symptom is painful cracks in the corner of the mouth. In cancer of oesophagus or stomach. Ulcers in mouth.

- CADMIUM SULPH.: When the patient feels chilly even near the fire, has nausea, vomiting. For cancer of throat, mouth or stomach.

There are many other medicines, only a few have been mentioned here.

ANAEMIA (DEFICIENCY OF BLOOD)

There are two kinds of cells in the blood, red and white. When the percentage of red blood cells is reduced we call it anaemia. It is due to loss of blood in menses, piles or injuries. Sometimes, it occurs due to grief, sorrow, mental worries or malnutrition.

- CHINA 3 or 6: When it is due to loss of blood.
- CALCAREA PHOS. 12X: In all kinds of anaemia, 5 grains or 5 tablets twice daily dry or with milk.
- FERRUM MUR. 3X TRIT.: Specially suited to women. 4 grains dry on tongue after meals.
- PULS.: For new cases, suits women.
- NATRUM MUR. 30, 200: For chronic cases due to emotional or psychological disorders.
- ARS A. 3X: When there is extreme prostration and restlessness.
- NATRUM SULPH. 6X: For bilious patients.
- FERRUM ARS 3X TRIT., PICRIC ACID, FERRUM MET. and PHOS. are also indicated.

RHEUMATISM, GOUT ETC.

Rheumatism, Gout, Arthritis, Sciatica, Lumbago, Synovitis etc. are diseases of one group and pain is the prominent symptom in them. Sometimes the pain is in the back, sometimes in joint or nerve or muscle.

Rheumatic pain can be either in muscles or joints, and in joints there is sometimes swelling also. Pain in joints with subacute swelling is termed. Lumbago is the name given to pain in back-lumbar region. Pain and swelling of knees etc. is called Synovitis. Sciatica is the pain of sciatic nerve which starts from lower back and goes right up to the foot.

Here are a few medicines which cure all these different pains if symptoms tally.

- ACONITE 3x, 30: In acute pains with swelling and fever, restlessness, urine highly coloured. Specially useful when due to exposure to dry cold wind. May be repeated every 2-3 hours till fever and pain subside.
- BRYONIA: The general character of the pain here is stitching and tearing, which gets worse by least motion, better by rest. Constipation, thirst, swelling and pains mostly right-sided. A dose of low potency often cures right sided Sciatica, Synovitis or Rheumatism.
- RHUS TOX.: Pains worse during rest, better when in motion and during hot-fomentation. Restlessness, worse by cold wind, rainy and cloudy season. Specific for lumbago. Often the pain is felt when the patient begins to move but is relieved by continuous motion.
- LAC CANINUM: Erratic pains, changing side alternately is an important symptom. Sciatica right side. Cramps in feet, legs feel numb and stiff, burning in palms and soles.
- LACNANTHES: Pain in neck, stiffness of neck, neck drawn to one side, chilliness between the shoulder blades.
- COLCHICUM Q or 30: Acute rheumatic pains. Swelling or no swelling, the painful spot turns white when pressed with finger. Stitching pain, worse in night, backache, joints stiff, gout, pain worse in warm weather. feverish, pain changing place.
- APIS: Thirst less, oedematous swelling of painful parts, worse in heat, urine scanty, stinging pain. Synovitis.

- PULSATILLA: Shifting pains in joints, thirst less, worse on letting limbs hang down. Weeping mood, worse in heat, lying on painless side, better in open air, slow motion and cold.
- CIMICIFUGA: Muscular soreness and pain in chest, back calves, etc. better in heat.
- CAULOPHYLLUM: Small joints of arms and legs, pains shift location.
- CALCAREA FLOUR. 6X: Backache, worse after rest, better while in gentle motion, worse in damp weather, relieved by fomentation and rubbing.
- BERBERIS: Lumbago, scanty urine, nausea, gall stone or stone in kidneys. Give mother tincture 5 drops in hot water three or four times a day.

SCIATICA

Pain affecting the back, hip, and outer side of the leg, caused by compression of a spinal nerve root in the lower back, often owing to degeneration of an intervertebral disc.

- AMMONIUM MUR.: Pain worse while sitting, somewhat better on moving but completely relieved on lying down.
- COLOCYNTH: Excruciating pain, mostly on the left side, better on putting pressure and heat, numbness with pain, pain right thigh, cramp-like pain in hip.
- GNAPHALIUM: Pain mostly on left side, cramps in calves and legs, anterior cranial neuralgia, numbness alternates with pain. Intense pain along the Sciatic nerve.
- LYCOPODIUM: Right-sided pain, worse between 4 p.m. and 8 p.m.
- MAGNESIA PHOS. 3X, 6X: Electric pain, relieved by heat. Immediate relief can be obtained by giving with hot water frequently.
- LEDUM: Gouty pain which begins with toe and travels upwards.

- SULPHUR: In chronic cases, when indicated remedies do not seem to act.
- SPIGELIA: Left-sided Sciatica.
- BRYONIA: Right-sided Sciatica.

PARALYSIS

When movement of any part or whole of the body is retarded, we call it Paralysis. Sometimes single parts are affected such as tongue, eyes, speech, hand, leg, etc., while at other times half of the body is involved.

- ACONITE: In acute cases when some part or whole of the body is affected and it is due to exposure to dry cold winds.
- CONIUM: In paralysis of old persons. Heavy legs.
- CAUSTICUM: Head remedy. Has cured many cases. Right-sided Hemiplegia. Paralysis of vocal cords, worse in dry cold winds, better in damp weather.
- GELSEMIUM: Jerking, cramps, electric current-like pain, eye lids fall, ptosis.
- OLEANDER: Painless paralysis.
- LATHYRUS: Staggering, paralysis of legs.
- CURARE: Muscular paralysis, impairing of sensation and consciousness. Paralysis of respiratory muscles.
- AGARICUS: Trembling, jerking.
- BARYTA CARB: Paralysis of half face.
- PLUMBUM: Obstinate constipation, paralysis of a single muscle.
- OPIUM: Unable to pass urine or stool.
- LACHESIS: Left-sided constriction of throat.
- AURUM MET.: High blood pressure. General Paralysis. Anguish.

18

DISEASES OF THE WOMEN

There are some special organs in women which are meant for conception, development and birth of the child. These are vagina, womb or uterus, ovaries, fallopian tubes and mammae (breasts). The diseases of these generative organs are commonly known as diseases of women. Treatment of these is briefly given hereunder.

VAGINITIS

Inflammation of the vagina.

- ACONITE 3X: When there is fever with chill, restlessness, inflammation and burning in vagina, urination difficult.
- ARNICA: For inflammation due to injury.
- CANTHARIS: When there is burning and pain in urine.
- MERCURIUS: To be used after Aconite when pus is formed.
- SEPIA: When the trouble is due to gonorrhoea, with tearing down sensation as if all the organs will fall out of the vagina. Itching and pus.
- BORAX: When there is profuse pus.
- NITRIC ACID: When it is due to abuse of mercury.
- SULPHUR: For fistulous ulcer in vagina, itching, burning.

- DULCIS: When there is much itching which gets worse in the night, jaundice and white motions.
- STAPHYSAGRIA: When there is pain during coition.
- ARSENIC: When there are watery eruptions, burning, restlessness, septic conditions.

PUERPERAL FEVER OR SEPTIC FEVER

Sometimes septic fever occurs after childbirth. It is due to some infection during labour such as handling the case with unwashed hands, using dirty linen, or due to retention of a piece of placenta. Fever is high and often fatal, if not treated properly. Medical aid should be given immediately in such cases.

- PYROGEN., VERATRUM VIR., BELL., KALI CYAN. and RHUS TOX. are some of the important remedies.

STERILITY

When sufficient time has passed after marriage and the woman is not suffering from any disease but she does not conceive, she is said to be sterile. But before declaring her sterile, the husband's semen should be examined. If no defect is found with the man, the woman should be treated for Sterility.

- CONIUM: It is the head remedy. Late and scanty menses. Pain in breasts before or during menses. 30 or 200 potency should be given once a week for a long time.
- BORAX 6 or 30: For those who suffer from Leucorrhoea.
- IODIUM: If breasts shrink or are undeveloped.
- SEPIA: When desire is diminished or absent. Indifference to the loved ones.
- PHOS.: When desire is increased, there is bleeding from nose.
- AGNUS CASTUS, BAR. M., GRAPHITES, MEDORRHINUM, NATRUM MUR., PLATINA and SABAL SER. are also useful.

HYSTERIA

This is also mostly a disease of women, in men it is found as an exception. It is connected with the generative organs of women. Some classify it with marital diseases. The patient generally becomes unconscious or remains semi-conscious. When camphor or some fragrant substance is smelt or cold water is sprinkled on the face, consciousness returns. But drastic measures should not be taken to bring the Patient back to consciousness.

- IGNATIA: Head remedy. A ball rises from the stomach and chokes the throat, silent brooding, sad and then joyful, the patient conceals facts. Fits due to grief, sorrow or any emotion.
- PLATINA: When there is sadness, restlessness. The patient tells about her disease to everybody. She is arrogant, proud, has contempt for others.
- ASAFOETIDA: When there is flatulence and spasmodic contraction of the stomach, ball in the throat.
- VALERIANA Q: When there are frequent fits, the patient is nervous, peevish, flatulence. This remedy sometimes acts well when well selected medicines fail.
- NUX MOSCHATA, NUX V., CIMICIFUGA, PULS., TARENTULA are some other indicated drugs.

ABORTION

- SABINA: When abortion is threatened in the first three months, i.e. pain starts and a discharge appears, this medicine should be given every 2 hours. In cases of habitual abortions in the first three months, weekly doses of 30 potency should be given.
- ARNICA: When abortion is threatened due to lifting a heavy weight or any sort of injury.

- SECALE: When abortion is threatened in the 4th or 5th month.
- CHAMOMILLA: When the cause is some mental excitement or anger.
- PULS. 200 or SECALE 200: One or two doses should be given after abortion.
- ALETRIS FARINOSA Q: 5 drops twice daily during pregnancy should be given to those who habitually abort again and again.

MENSTRUAL DISEASES

From the age of 12-13 until 45-50 every women has her menses from 3 to 5 days regularly. Irregularity in the course results in diseases of which brief treatment is given as under.

AMENORRHOEA

An abnormal absence of menstruation.

- PULSATILLA: This is called the women's remedy. It covers many ailments of women. If menses do not appear between the age of 12 to 14 this remedy will help. Its characteristic symptom is lateness — everything is too late. First flow does not appear in time or monthly course is always late not only by days and weeks but sometimes by months. On account of late and scanty menses many symptoms appear, such as heaviness of head, loss of appetite, nausea, chillness, leucorrhoea, palpitation, anaemia, etc. This remedy relieves all these symptoms. Patient is mild. tearful.
- SULPHUR: In chronic cases of amenorrhoea.
- SENECIO Q: When even the first menstrual flow has not appeared or suppressed after one or two flows, 2-3 drops should be given for a few days. It is a good remedy for irregular menses. Sometimes after suppression of menses

bleeding from nose or mouth starts and symptoms of T.B. appear. It will relieve all such symptoms. Give 2-3 drops twice or thrice daily.

- ACONITE: If suppression of menses is due to cold.
- BRYONIA: When there is stitching pain, cough, blood from nose and mouth in places of menses.
- CIMICIFUGA: When there are no menses, pain in pelvic region, mostly on the left side.
- FERRUM MET.: When amenorrhoea in due to anaemia, it should be given in alternation with PULS.
- MANGANESE DIOXIDE 1X: Suppressed menses reappear by giving one grain dose 3-4 times a day. Hot fomentation. is useful.
- CONIUM: For irregular menses that occur in two, three or four months.
- CHINA: When there is debility resulting in suppression of menses.
- HAMAMELIS: When there is bleeding from nose and mouth in place of menses.
- FERRUM PHOS.: When the nose bleeds.
- SEPIA: When there is a scanty flow.
- GRAPHITES: When there is itch in vagina, late menses Suits fat women.

DYSMENORRHOEA

Painful menstruation, typically involving abdominal cramps.

- PULSATILLA: For late and scanty flow, when there is pain in back and pelvic region; dark, thick discharge.
- CIMICIFUGA: When there is headache before menses, pain extends to thighs. Dark, scanty discharge.
- BELLADONNA: When there is headache, pain one day before the flow starts, pain with the feeling as if all the parts will protrude out and fall down.
- MAGNESIA PHOS. 3X TRIT.: 5 grains dissolved in hot water

every 15 or 30 minutes will relieve severe pains. Hot fomentation on lower abdomen and back is sedative.

- APIS: When there is stinging pain.
- CAULOPHYLLUM: When there is spasmodic and stitching pain and it extends to other parts of the body. During pain mother tincture be given 3-4 times a day.
- XANTHOXYLUM, COCCULUS, CHAMOMILLA GELS., SEPIA and SECALE should also be consulted.

MENORRHAGIA

Abnormally heavy bleeding at menstruation.

- ASHOKA Q: This is said to be the best medicine for excessive flow. 4 to 5 drops to be given twice daily for some time.
- CALCAREA CARB.: Suited to fat women. When there is an early profuse and protracted flow.
- CHINA: When there is ringing in ears and debility due to excessive dark discharge.
- HYDRASTIS 1 or 3X: For all sorts of profuse menses. Give for some time twice or thrice daily.
- SABINA: When there is red blood, suits bulky ladies.
- CROCUS SAT.: When there is black, clotty, offensive discharge.
- HAMAMELIS: When there is a dark discharge or bleeding due to injury or strain.
- MILLEFOLIUM: When there is profuse red blood.
- THLASPI BURSA PASTORIS Q: 4-5 drops twice daily for painful, profuse, long standing flow.
- FICUS RELIGIOSA Q: In all kinds of menorrhagia.
- ERIGERON Q: When there is irritation in rectum, bright red flow, gets worse on the least motion.
- BORAX, CHAMOMILLA, PLATINA and FERRUM should also be studied.

LEUCORRHOEA

A whitish or yellowish discharge of mucus from the vagina.

- PULSATILLA: Head remedy, when there is a yellowish, thick discharge.
- CALCAREA CARB.: When there is milky discharge with burning and itching.
- SEPIA: When there is yellow greenish discharge which is offensive. Suited to thin women.
- NITRIC ACID: In old cases, cases due to abuse of mercury, when there is an offensive discharge.
- ALUMINA: When there is burning, profuse watery discharge, which drops down to heels, the patient has constipation, gets better with cold.
- AMBRA G.: When it gets worse in the night, has a mucus discharge, stitching pain.
- BORAX: When it is white like white of eggs with a sensation as if hot water was flowing, makes woman nervous, she cannot bear noise.
- BOVISTA: When there is a thick, slimy discharge, yellow stains on linen, increased sexual desire, excoriating discharge which gets worse on motion. The patient thinks her head has become bigger.
- GRAPHITES: When there is thin, excoriating discharge which gets worse in the morning on rising. Suits fat women, there is hardness of uterus and ovaries.
- KREOSOTE: When the flow stains linen, yellowish discharges, produces ulcers.
- SULPHUR: In chronic cases.

CLIMAX

At the age of about 45 the monthly course in women stops permanently, and this period is called Climacteric period or

Climax. These days menses are often prolonged for many days, the discharge is profuse and the patient becomes weak and anaemic. Medicines mentioned under Menorrhagia should be used. In addition to them, the following medicines have been found efficacious.

- LACHESIS: It is the best remedy for diseases of this period. Use it when there is profuse discharge, burning in palms, burning on the head, sweating, which get worse after sleep.
- SANGUINARIA 3X: When there is a profuse flow, the patient feels as if everything will fall down, and as if the vagina has become large.
- JABORANDI: When there is profuse sweating and restlessness.

DISEASES OF THE UTERUS

METRITIS

Inflammation of the uterus.

- VERATRUM VIRIDE 3X: This medicine has proved useful in the first stage of inflammation of the uterus. It relieves pain, fever, chill, nearly all the symptoms.
- PYROGENIUM 30, 200: To be used in later stages when there is offensive pus and septic conditions set in.
- SABINA: When there is a discharge of red blood or clotted blood.
- BELLADONNA: When there is pain, burning, the patient feels as if all the organs will come out of the vagina.
- HYDRASTIS Q: When there is burning in the neck of uterus, thick yellowish discharge.
- SEPIA: In chronic cases, when there is a bearing down feeling, itch, scanty discharge.

DISPLACEMENT (FLEXIONS OR VERSIONS)

Sometimes the uterus looses its erect position and bends forward or backward or becomes loose and comes down.

- SEPIA: It is the best medicine. The patient presses her parts with the hand so that the organs may not fall out. There is a constant bearing down feeling.
- AURUM MURIATICUM NATRONATUM: In many cases, this medicine is indicated, specially in chronic cases and prolapsus when the uterus comes out of the vagina, also when the uterus has gone hard, there are ulcers in the vagina or the neck of uterus.
- ARNICA: When the trouble is due to injury or accident.
- AURUM MET.: When this happens after lifting heavy weight.
- FRAXINUS: For atonic conditions of uterus.
- FERRUM IOD 3X, BELL., CIMICIFUGA and LILIUM TIG. should also be tried.

In this disease an experienced nurse or lady doctor would set the fallen or prolapsed womb right by manipulation and if necessary a rubber ring is placed inside to keep the uterus in position. After sometime the ring is removed.

TUMOR OR CANCER

At the time of menopause, i.e. about the age between 40 and 50 a tumor or cancer develops in some women. An early detection and treatment with Homoeopathic remedies cures the disease.

- CALCAREA IODIDE 3X TRIT.: In all kinds of tumors give 2-3 grains 3 times a day dry on tongue.
- ARSENIC IOD. 3X: For cancer.
- CADMIUM SULPH.: This too is efficacious in cancer.

- CONIUM: In high and higher potencies it has cured tumors as well as cancers.
- THUJA: For cancers, tumors or any other growth in the uterus.
- RUTA Q: It is claimed that one drop of this medicine in sugar of milk given once a week or even two weeks will cure cancerous growth.
- CARCINOSIN 200, 1000: Usable in all cases once or twice a month with other remedies.
- THLASPI BURSA PASTORIS Q, HYDRASTIS Q and LACHESIS are also indicated.

DISEASES OF THE OVARIES

OVARITIS

- ACONITE: When accompanied with fever, restlessness, due to catching cold, with pain in urine.
- APIS: When there is stinging pain mostly on the right side, urine scanty, no thirst.
- LACHESIS: For left-sided pain when even the touch of clothes is unbearable, belt is not bearable.
- CONIUM: In chronic cases, in hardness of ovaries.
- THUJA: For hardness of the left side, chronic cases, the patient feels better on hot fomentation.
- AURUM MURIATICUM NATRONATUM, PLATINA, GRAPHITES, PULS., COLOCYNTH, FERRUM PHOS. should also he consulted.

DROPSY OF THE OVARIES

- APIS: For right-sided dropsy, when there is stinging pain, fluid collects in ovary, it is swollen and sometimes pus is also formed.

- IODIUM: For the right ovary when there is a bearing down feeling, pain and collection of fluid. Medicines under ovaries be tried.

OVARALGIA

Neuralgic pain in the ovaries.

- NAJA: Chief remedy, when there is severe pain without swelling or inflammation.
- ATROPIA 3X: For immediate relief during pain.
- MAGNESIA PHOS. 3X: For immediate relief take 5 grains or 5 tablets dissolved in hot water frequently.
- ZINCUM VALERIANA, STAPHISAGRIA and COLOCYNTH are also used.

Tumor or Cancer

- LACHESIS, KREOSOTE, ARS, AURUM MUR. NAT. are chief remedies.
- BELL., CALCAREA, SEPIA, LYCO, APIS and IODIUM are useful for right ovary. For left ovary LACHESIS, LILIUM, KALI CARB., STRAMONIUM and NAJA are indicated.
- CONIUM has been useful in chronic cases.

DISEASES OF MAMMAE

The breasts of women are regarded as generative organs. When the ovaries are affected the disease is reflected in mammae.

MASTODYNIA

Pain in the breasts.

- CONIUM: Head remedy. When there is pain in both the breasts before menses, hardness, scanty menses.

- SANGUINARIA: When there is pain in the right breast which gets worse on deep breathing.
- CIMICIFUGA: For the left breast.
- CALCAREA CARB.: When there is pain about a week before menses, profuse flow.
- PULS.: When there is pain in both the breasts, menses scanty.

ABSCESS OR SWELLING

- BELLADONNA: When the breasts are red, there is swelling, and pain due to injury, in a nursing mother.
- ACONITE: When it is due to cold with fever and pain.
- BRYONIA: When there is hardness and a tendency to formation of abscess.
- HEPAR: If pus is formed.
- CALC. SULPH.: After the abscess opens and pus comes out, it will heal up.
- SILICEA and PHYTOLACCA are also useful.

TUMOR OR CANCER

- PHYTOLACCA: Chief remedy.
- CONIUM: This has cured many cases of tumors and cancer.
- Other remedies — HYDRASTIS, ARS, CIMICIFUGA, THUJA, ARS., IOD.

NIPPLES' DISEASES

BURNING AND ITCHING

AGARICUS, ARS and SULPHUR.

CRACKS, FISSURES

CUNDURANGO, CONIUM, GRAPHITES, PHYT., SIL.

RETRACTION

SILICEA, SARSAPARILLA, HYDRASTIS.

PAIN, SORENESS AND TENDERNESS

In addition to remedies already mentioned under different heads, please study LAC CAN. (dries up milk), CIM., RAN. B., LAPIS, CROT T.

19

DISEASES OF THE CHILDREN

There are a few diseases that effect only children and only those diseases are mentioned in this chapter. All other diseases mentioned in preceding chapters can attack children also and they can be treated by the medicines mentioned in respective cases.

INFANTILE LIVER

At the time of birth the liver of the baby extends by a few inches in the abdomen and during the first two months it reduces to its normal size below the ribs. But sometimes this process is retarded and the liver remains enlarged in the abdomen. The baby gets indigestion and diarrhoea, jaundice sets in and water accumulates in the abdomen. There is oedematous swelling of face, hands and feet.

- CALCAREA ARS 3X: Chief remedy.
- CHAMOMILLA: To be given if jaundice sets in the first week itself of the birth.
- CALCAREA CARB.: If the child's head is large, there is sweat on head, abdomen bloated, whitish stools, diarrhoea.

- PODOPHYLLUM: When there are watery stools with all other symptoms.
- MERC. SOL.: When the eyes are yellowish.
- NITRIC ACID: When there are ulcers in the mouth.
- KALMEGH Q: This medicine is said to have cured many cases in drop doses twice or thrice daily.
- CHELIDONIUM Q: When the eyes are yellow, stools white.
- CARDUS Q: For chronic cases.

DISEASES OF THE NAVEL

After birth sometimes the navel is swollen and painful and sometimes pus is formed.

- CALENDULA Q: 10 drops to an ounce or two of hot water should be used to wash the navel and Calendula ointment should be applied.
- SILICEA 30: Should be given if there is pus.
- BELLADONNA: For simple swelling with redness and pain.
- ARS. A.: In offensive pus.

PROLAPSUS ANI

At the time of passing stool a portion of the rectum comes out of the anus.

- PODOPHYLLUM: Chief remedy.
- PHOS.: If some blood comes out.
- ACID MUR.: When it comes out even with urine.
- EQUISETUM Q or 6: For children who have dreams and nightmares.
- KREOSOTE: In dreams of urinating. Passes involuntarily during the first part of night.
- SULPHUR: In chronic cases.
- PULS. and SILICEA are also useful.

OPEN FONTANELLES

On the top of the head of the child there are two triangular portions, once near the forehead and the other in the same line 2 to 3 inches backward, which are soft at the time of the birth but within 3 to 4 months the bones are formed and they become hard. But sometimes this process is delayed and is harmful.

- SULPHUR 30: Once a week will do. But if it fails give CALCAREA CARB. 30 once a week for a few weeks.
- CALCAREA PHOS. and SILICEA are also needed sometimes.

ULCERS IN THE MOUTH

- BORAX 3X TRIT.: The best remedy in white ulcers.
- RHUS TOX. and VIOLA TRICOLOR are also indicated.

LICE IN THE HEAD

- SABADILLA Q: Its lotion 1 to 20 should be used to wash the head.
- NATRUM MUR. 12X and STAPHYSAGRIA should be tried internally.

HYDROCEPHALUS

A condition in which fluid accumulates in the brain, typically in young children, enlarging the head and sometimes causing brain damage.

- SULPHUR, CALCAREA and SILICEA should be given according to symptoms.

DENTITION

During dentition one or the other malady always troubles the child.

- CHAMOMILLA 6: The best remedy if the child is peevish and has green and yellow watery stools.
- FERRUM PHOS. 6X: If there is fever and cold.
- CALCAREA PHOS. 6X: Dentition will be much easier if 2 to 3 grains of this medicine are given daily to the child.

ENURESIS

Involuntary urination, especially by children at night.

- CINA: When the child does not awaken even after passing urine and has worms.
- BELLADONNA: When the child urinates during deep sleep.
- GELS.: When even during the day the urge is imperative.
- ACID BENZOIC: When the urine is offensive.
- LYCO: If Uric Acid is found in urine.
- VERBASCUM Q (MULLEIN OIL): 3-4 drops twice daily are found to be very useful.
- FERRUM PHOS. 6X, 200X: Daily or weekly are very efficacious.
- SEPIA and SULPHUR should also be studied.

MARASMUS

In this disease the child looses flesh, eats much but the food is not assimilated. Abdomen is enlarged but hands and feet become very thin.

- SULPHUR 30: Begin the treatment with SULPHUR 30 and after a few days give CALCAREA CARB. 30 for some time.

- ABROTANUM: The chief remedy of this disease.
- IODIUM: When the child has a voracious appetite.
- CALCAREA CARB. is useful for fatty children who have weak bones and a lack of calcium. For thin and lean children CALCAREA PHOS. should be given.

WEEPING

When the child weeps without any apparent cause, the following medicines may be given.

- CHAMOMILLA: When the child is very irritable he cries, wants to be carried in the lap, weeps again as soon as one stops moving.
- JALAPA: When the child sleeps in the day and weeps at night.
- LYCO: When the child weeps in the day and sleeps in the night.
- IGNATIA: When the child trembles during weeping.
- CUPRUM: When the child behaves as if choking his respiration due to anger during weeping.
- PSORINUM: When the child weeps all day and night.

FOR DEVELOPMENT OF UNDERDEVELOPED CHILDREN

- AGARICUS: When the child learns to talk and walk late and often falls down when tries to walk.
- BARYTA CARB: For physical and mental development. Stunted growth, childish behaviour even in advanced age, the child does not want to play.
- CAL. PHOS. 6X: For late dentition, weak bones.
- LATHYRUS: For staggering, knees knock against each other while walking.

- ABROTANUM: When the neck is so weak that he cannot hold his head up. Legs greatly emaciated. Abdomen distended.

20

FIRST AID AND EMERGENCIES

There are occasions when one is suddenly injured, slightly or seriously, and needs to be provided immediate aid and care. In many cases one is more shocked than injured, and shock itself requires treatment.

There are burns, fainting, sting and bites, nose bleed, hiccups and fits, cramps in the night and various kinds of accidents. These should be provided the usual First Aid quickly and intelligently, till proper medical aid arrives. The patient should be moved to a suitable place and kept warm. If the skin is broken, the wound should be cleaned and covered. If artificial respiration is needed, it should be given. If poison has been swallowed, it should be emitted by vomiting. Medicines should be given as follows:

INJURIES

- ARNICA MONT.: It is the head remedy for injuries, falls, blows, contusions. It is specially suited to cases when any injury, however remote, seems to have caused the present troubles. It should be used internally in 30 or 200 potency.

Linen or lint soaked in its mother tincture should be packed locally on the swelling or injured part.

- CALENDULA: In injuries when the skin is ruptured. Its mother tincture is applied locally or the wound is drenched with its lotion (1 to 10). It promotes healthy granulation and heals even chronic wounds. It is used in ointment or lotion form in scalds, burns and even gangrenes.
- HYPERICUM: This is a recommended remedy for injuries to nerves, specially of fingers, toes and nails. Use it for crushed fingers, lips, punctured wounds. Relieves excessive pains after injury, injured nerves after animal bites, lacerated wounds with much prostration from loss of blood. Use tincture of 200 potency.
- SYMPHYTUM: It is the chief remedy of injuries to sinews, tendons or periosteum. Of great use in wounds penetrating to perineum and bones and in non-union of fractures, in irritable stump after amputation, irritable bone at point of fracture. In pricking pain and soreness of periosteum, pain in eye after a blow of an obtuse body. Mother tincture is generally used internally as well as externally. In chronic cases 200 or higher potencies may be used.
- RHUS TOX.: It is useful for sprains or ailment from strain on any joint or organ.
- RUTA: Follows RHUS TOX. well in sprains. In lameness after sprain is relieved, injured bruised bones, pains after eye strain. In injuries to eye, straining of tendons, and injuries to periosteum and cartilages. It is used internally and mother tincture is used externally, pure or in lotions.
- STAPHISAGRIA: For cuts by sharp instruments. Should be given internally to allay pains in 6, 30 potency and the cut should be dressed with its lotion (1 to 10). It relieves pain after extraction of tooth, heals lacerated tissues. To stop bleeding Alum dissolved in cold water is used for

dressing. ARNICA should not be applied on open wounds, CALENDULA should be used instead.

- HAMAMELIS: It stops bleeding, and is used for dressing bleeding wounds. To stop bleeding if an artery is cut, press hard on the side of the heart with the thumb and then put a hard bandage over it. In case a vein is cut, press hard or lie on the side away from the heart. Blood will be stopped, then dress with CALENDULA, HAMAMELIS or any other medicine as required.
- NATRUM SULPH.: In head injuries when the brain is involved, and the patient is not conscious and is restless, this remedy should be repeated twice or thrice daily. In chronic effects, higher potencies are used.
- ECHINACEA Q: This medicine has proved very useful in gangrenes, i.e. ulcers which become septic and refuse to heal. It should be used in drop doses internally and the ulcers should be dressed with its lotion.
- GUNPOWDER 3X TRIT.: Very useful for obstinate ulcers. 3 to 4 grains twice daily dry on tongue will do.

SHOCKS

A medical condition associated with a fall in blood pressure, caused by such events as loss of blood, burns, allergic reaction, or sudden emotional stress, and marked by cold, pallid skin, irregular breathing, rapid pulse, and dilated pupils.

- CAMPHOR Q: 3 to 4 drops should be given with a little sugar; can be repeated every half hour.
- VERATRUM ALBUM 6 or CARBO VEG. 6 is also useful in shocks. For after effects use ARNICA 200 or ARSENIC 200.

INSECT BITES

- In bites by bees, scorpion, fleas or other insects external application of CAMPHOR Q or kerosene oil or onion juice is useful. The sting should be removed and it should be dressed with CALENDULA. Garlic is said to be very efficacious in such bites and its juice should be applied.
- APIS MEL. 6: In swelling, pain etc. twice daily will do.
- LEDUM 6: For rat bites; twice daily.

It is said that for scorpion bites lukewarm salt lotion should be dropped in the opposite side ear of the patient, i.e. if the bite is on the left leg, salt lotion should be dropped in the right ear.

BURNS

When there is an ordinary burn on any single part of the body, dress it with lime water. The burnt place should be kept covered with wheat flour or lotion of CANTHARIS Q (1 to 10) should be applied and the part be kept dressed with it.

- CANTHARIS 6: Should be used internally twice daily. If cow dung is applied to the burnt place, it is said no blisters are formed and burning etc. is also relieved. When the clothes catch fire, one should not run away but should lie down at once. The burning clothes should be covered with a blanket. When the burns are deep and serious, hospitalisation is necessary.
- ACONITE 3X or ARSENIC A. 30: In fever, restlessness, burning, etc. Should be given internally according to symptoms.

TRAVEL SICKNESS

Some people have nausea, vomiting and vertigo when travelling in a ship, steamer, bus or train in hills and in air. Sipping of lemon, orange etc. gives relief. Lying down also relieves. Sometimes these symptoms persist even after the journey. The following medicines are useful:

- ANTIM TART. 6, 30: When there is pressure in the abdomen, nausea and vomit.
- COCCULUS 6, 30: It is the chief remedy. Have a small phial of globules and sip 3 to 4 globules during travel frequently.
- APOMORPHIA 6: When there is noise in ears with all other symptoms.
- NUX V. 30: When there is ringing in ears.
- STAPHISAGRIA: For vertigo and in cases where the smoke of cigarettes increases the trouble. When the abdomen feels loose.
- THERIDION: For seasickness. When there is nausea and vomiting while closing eyes and while in motion.
- SANICULA: When one craves cold drinks. In cases of nausea and vomiting while car riding. In nausea while looking up. In cases when water is vomited as soon as it is taken. A hot belt should be put on the abdomen.

SUN OR HEAT STROKE

There is fever, headache and restlessness. Onion is its best remedy, its juice should be given internally and should also be applied externally on hands and feet. Apply cold water pack or ice bag on the head. Massage in the back bone with linen soaked in ice cold water is also useful.

- GLONOINE 6: It is the chief remedy if the fever is high. Should be repeated 1 to 2 hourly.

- BELLADONNA 3X: When there is high fever, severe headache, red face, red eyes.
- GELSEMIUM 3X, 6: When there is an absence of thirst, in high fever, prostration.
- NATRUM CARB.: In headaches during summer, or in its aggravation from sun, when one is sensitive to heat.
- NATRUM MUR.: In chronic cases, when there is fever and headache, etc. from 11 a.m. to 5p.m. For bilious patients.
- VERATRUM VIR. 3: When there is high fever, congestion in chest. It can be given every 15 minutes or so according to urgency.

III

CHARACTERISTICS OF SOME IMPORTANT MEDICINES

21

IMPORTANT MEDICINES

In the foregoing chapters though medicines for different diseases have been described yet in Homoeopathy the names of the diseases do not matter; it is the symptoms of the diseases that are to be tallied with the symptoms of the drugs. The drug which has symptoms closest to the symptoms of the disease is likely to cure it best.

In patients you will find that some symptoms are peculiar and therefore rather important. For example, a patient has fever, and fever is a common symptom in many cases, but with fever he has unquenchable thirst for small quantities of water, i.e., he drinks only a little but demands again after a few minutes. This is a peculiar and therefore important symptom of the patient, which is not found in all cases of fever. This symptom will not be found in all the medicines. These symptoms are called the characteristics of that particular medicine and if these characteristics symptoms tally, the medicine will surely relieve the patient, whatever the name of the disease. Given below are characteristic symptoms of 40 important medicines. When prescribing a medicine for a patient these symptoms should be kept in mind. For example, if a patient is thirstless he will not require ARSENIC. It is the same for other cases.

ACONITE

- Terrible anguish and fear of death, there is extreme restlessness and tossing about.
- Complaints brought about by exposure to dry cold winds or from a sudden checking of perspiration.
- Hard, full, fast pulse.
- The disease get worse in the evening and night, the attack is sudden and violent.

ANTIM TART.

- Large accumulation of mucus in chest, oppression of chest, rattling, wheezing.
- Difficult raising of phlegm, vomiting and drowsiness.
- Eruptions, pustules resembling those of small pox.

ANTIM CRUD.

- Thick milky white coating on the tongue. Fretful, peevish disposition, child cannot bear to be touched or even being looked at.
- Worse on bathing and in heat.
- Hard warts.
- Vomits soon after eating or drinking.

ARSENIC ALBUM

- Periodicity in disease. Fever etc. at a particular time.
- Weakness and prostration after slightest exertion.
- Malignity of symptoms.
- Restlessness and anguish.
- Burning all over the body.
- Pains get worse while resting at night and with cold.
- Unquenchable thirst for small quantities of water at short intervals.

ARNICA

- A bruised sore feeling all over the body, the patient feels as if he has been pounded.
- Useful in injuries.

APIS

- Drowsiness.
- Oedematous swelling.
- Thirstlessness
- Intolerance of heat.
- Stinging pains.
- Aggravation in the afternoon.
- Bruised sensations.

BAPTISIA

- Specific for typhoid fevers.
- Septic conditions of blood.
- Good for muscular soreness, offensive breath, stool, urine, sweat.

BARYTA CARB.

- Bashful, childish aversion to strangers.
- Tendency to catch cold easily.
- Tonsilitis.
- Mentally and physically backward.

BELLADONNA

- Pains gradually increase, suddenly decline and appear elsewhere.
- Painful shots that get sore on gentle pressure, yet firm pressure is tolerated.

- Hot, red skin, flushed face, full, hard pulse, throbbing carotids, delirium and hyperaesthesia (excessive sensitiveness) of the senses.
- Dilation of the pupils, photophobia and infected eyes.
- It affects mostly the right side of the body.

BRYONIA

- Apathy, ranging from languor to torpor.
- Relief from rest, aggravation from motion.
- Sharp, stitching pains.
- Warmth gives relief in all conditions except headache and eye symptoms.
- Pressure or lying on the painful side gives relief.

CANTHARIS

- Raw burning pains.
- Intolerable constant urging to urinate.
- Head remedy for burns.
- Worse on taking coffee.

COLOCYNTH

- Agonising abdominal colic relieved by bending double and pressing hard.
- Suitable for irritable, easily angered persons and ill effects therefrom.
- Sciatica better when pressure is added and in heat.

CALCAREA CARB.

- Fair, fat, flabby body.
- Sweat about the head.
- Large abdomen, great head, small neck.
- Cold feet, as if damp stockings were on.

- Sour vomiting.
- Diarrhoea with acid stomach, worse in the evening.
- Short breath.
- Slow, stupid, sluggish.
- Premature, profuse, protracted menses.

CHINA

- Sense of satiety after a few mouthfuls of food.
- Diseases due to loss of vital fluids — blood, semen, diarrhoea, polyuria. etc.
- Better in a warm room but increase of bleeding is relieved by cold air.
- Periodicity.
- Indigestion, flatulence.

CHAMOMILLA

- Crossness, irritability, the child wants to be carried in lap, otherwise cries.
- Intolerance of pain.
- Worse in warmth, in the evening and night.

CARBO VEG.

- Discharges offensive.
- Putridity and burning.
- Coldness of legs and knees.
- Flatulence, eructations.
- Venous sluggishness, even stagnation.

DULCAMARA

- Ailments due to being drenched in rain.
- Worse in cold, damp weather or a sudden change of temperature from hot to cold.

- Irritable.

GELSEMIUM

- Dull, stupid, apathetic mental condition.
- Great weakness, muscular relaxation and deep seated aching.
- Paralytic action on muscles of the eyes.
- Light thirstless fever.
- Complaints arising from emotional disturbances.
- Stage fright, apprehension.

GRAPHITES

- Fatty, clubby, costive, eczema, dry as well as wet.
- Scabby eruptions.
- Music makes are weep, every little injury suppurates.

HEPAR SULPH.

- Suppurative (pus producing) tendency.
- Sensitive to cold air.
- Oversensitiveness of nervous system.
- Craving for strong things, as acids etc.
- Unhealthy skin, every little would suppurates.

IGNATIA

- Chief remedy of Hysteria, ailments from grief, worry, disappointment, mortification etc.
- Silent brooding.
- Superficial and erratic character of symptoms.

IPECAC.

- Constant nausea, even after vomit.

- Clean tongue.
- Dry spasmodic cough.

KALI BICHROM.

- Tenacious, stingy expectoration.
- Ulcers which tend to perforate.
- Troubles of fat, fair, chubby children.
- Painful spots that can be covered under finger tip.
- Post nasal catarrh.

LYCOPODIUM

- Aggravation from 4 to 8 p.m.
- Complaints travel from right to left.
- Worse from cold.
- Offensiveness of discharge, red sediment in urine.

LACHESIS

- Great sensitiveness of body and intolerance of clothing around the neck.
- Remedy for the left side.
- General aggravation after sleep, the patients sleeps with aggravation.
- Useful in climacteric disorders.
- General blueness of the skin and eruptions.

NUX VOM.

- Thin, spare, irascible patients of nervo-bilious temperament, with great sensitiveness to external impressions.
- Ailments brought out by drastic medicines, purgatives, sedentary habits, rich food, etc.
- Tired, worn out feeling in the morning or on waking.

- Constipation.

MERC. COR.

- Dysentery with blood and pain and tenseness.
- Worse at night, better during rest.

MERC. SOL.

- Fetid breath.
- Flabby tongue showing imprint of teeth.
- External soreness of the throat.
- Sensitiveness to cold air.
- Superficial character of ulcerations.
- Soreness of the right side.
- Straining, 'never got done' feeling at stools.
- Easy respiration.
- Nocturnal aggravation.

NATRUM MUR.

- Malnutrition, emaciation and anaemia.
- Hammering in the frontal region of the head.
- Eruptions on the margin of hairy scalp.
- Backache which gets better by lying on something hard. Violent thirst.
- Aversion to bread.
- Worse from 11 a.m. to 5p.m.

PHOSPHORUS

- Fatty degeneration of tissues.
- Caries of bones.
- Dread of mental exertion.
- Painless diarrhoea with exhaustion and prostration.
- Low grade fever with absence of thirst.

- Oppression of chest.
- Burning pain in the dorsal region of spine.
- Stumbling when walking and trembling of legs.
- Worse on lying on the left side.
- The patient likes ice-cold water.

PHOSPHORIC ACID

- Debility from nervous causes.
- Painless, watery, exhausting diarrhoea.
- Ailments from sexual excess.
- Pain on vertex as if crushed.

PULSATILLA

- Tearfulness, mild, gentle, yielding disposition, changeableness and fickleness of symptoms.
- Worse in the evening, after eating and during rest.
- Relief from motion and in cool open air.
- Paleness of face and chilliness, even with a sensation of heat.
- All discharges are bland in character and yellow or
- yellowish green.
- Thirstlessness.
- Everything occurs too late, coryza in late stages, indigestion two hours after eating, menses never in time.

RHUS TOX.

- Extreme restlessness, the patient changes side and place every few minutes.
- Relief from motion, aggravation from rest.
- Worse in cold and damp and rainy season.
- Headache as if a board were strapped on the forehead.
- Aching in occipital (back of head) protuberances.
- White coated tongue but the tip is red.

SULPHUR

- Dirty and poor habits of the body.
- Aversion to water and washing.
- A sinking feeling in the stomach about 11 a.m.
- "Catnap" sleep.
- Heat at the top of the head and burning of palms and soles.
- Defective reaction after carefully selected remedies fail to act.
- Stooping walk.
- Drinks much, eats little.
- Morning diarrhoea which drives the patient out of the bed.
- Nocturnal aggravation.

SILICEA

- Ulcers or fistula or abscesses which refuse to heal.
- Offensive foot sweat.
- Constipation-stool comes out with difficulty, when partly expelled, it recedes back.
- Headache which begins from the neck and extends to the eyes.
- Aggravation from cold, at new moon and in the morning.

SPONGIA

- Heart and throat affections.
- Anxiety and difficult breathing.
- Exhaustions and heaviness of the body after slightest exertion.
- Swelling and pain in testicles.

SPIGELIA

- Left-sided remedy, Hemicrania left-sided, sun headache.
- Sciatica-Neuralgia.
- Great Heart remedy.

SEPIA

- Women's remedy. Bearing down sensation as if everything would escape through Vulva.
- Indifferent to those loved best.
- Worse on washing or in dampness.
- Better during exercise and warmth.

THUJA

- Head remedy for warts, vaccinosis.
- Music causes weeping.
- A feeling as if soul and body were separated.
- Great antimycotic.

VERATRUM ALBUM

- Cold sweats, body cold, burning internally.

22

MEDICINES FOR YOUR HOME

Here are some of the important medicines for your family chest. You may buy them gradually. The ones noted earlier are required more often; those noted later are needed in special cases only.

1. Aconite Napellus
2. Arsenicum Album
3. Belladonna
4. Bryonia Alba
5. Ipecac
6. Nux Vomica
7. Pulsatilla
8. Hepar Sulph.
9. Lycopodium
10. Mercurius Sol.
11. Chamomilla
12. Sulphur
13. China
14. Arnica Mont.
15. Rhus Tox.
16. Antim. Tart.
17. Antim. Crud.
18. Cantharis

19. Carbo Veg.
20. Cuprum Met.
21. Veratrum Album
22. Cina
23. Apis Mel.
24. Phosphorus
25. Mercurius Cor.
26. Gelsemium
27. Lachesis
28. Acid. Phos.
29. Acid. Hydro.
30. Acid. Nitric.
31. Colocynth
32. Opium
33. Terebinthina
34. Baptisia
35. Calcarea Carb.
36. Cimicifuga
37. Sepia
38. Silicea
39. Ignatia
40. Natrum Mur.
41. Dulcamara
42. Drosera
43. Coffea
44. Stramonium
45. Kali Bichrom.
46. Kali Carb.
47. Baryta Carb.
48. Graphites
49. Naja (Cobra)
50. Veratrum Vir.
51. Digitalis
52. Cannabis Indica
53. Cannabis Sativa
54. Cicuta Vir.

55. Hamamelis
56. Hyoscyamus
57. Cocculus Indicus
58. Euphrasia
59. Podophyllum
60. Sabina
61. Secale Cor.
62. Spigelia
63. Spongia
64. Colchicum
65. Aethusa Cyn.
66. Calendula
67. Thuja
68. Conium Mac.
69. Eupatorium Perf.
70. Iris Ver.
71. Staphisagria
72. Tabacum
73. Hydrastis
74. Chininum Sulph.
75. Platina
76. Sabadilla
77. Anacardium
78. Nux Moschata
79. Rheum
80. Sambucus
81. Rhododendron
82. Rananculus Bulb.
83. Teucrium
84. Kreosotum
85. Leptandra
86. Cuprum Aceticum
87. Croton Tig.
88. Caulophyllum
89. Aurum Met.
90. Aloe Socotrina

91. Plumbum
92. Cactus G.
93. Dioscorea
94. Ferrum Phos.
95. Kali Mur.
96. Calcarea Phos.
97. Kali Phos.
98. Natrum Phos.
99. Natrum Sulph.
100. Magnesia Phos.
101. Calcarea Flour
102. Agaricus
103. Ruta
104. Calcarea Sulph.

SOME MEDICINES IN MOTHER TINCTURE

1. Arnica
2. Calendula
3. Hamamelis
4. Hydrastis
5. Camphor
6. Cedron
7. Thuja
8. Blatta Q

Wooden family chests and pocket cases of 12, 24, 48, 104 or more medicines are available from all Homoeopathic chemists. It is better to have a chest of about 100 phials but in the beginning one may purchase only 30, 40 medicines. Other medicines can be purchased as and when required. Thus gradually the box will be full and the medicines will be the ones that you need in the family. Some medicines should be purchased both in lower and higher potentices — e.g. 30 as well as 200. One may otherwise have lower potencies only in the beginning like, 6 and 30.

The box to be purchased should have the capacity of holding 2 dram phials, so that though ordinarily you may order one dram medicine, when you need any 2 dram medicines they may also be accommodated.

As regards the procedure of dispensing medicine we have already given it in detail in the first chapter. A drop of liquid medicine put in an ounce of water can be divided into 2 doses for adults and 4 for children. Similarly, a drop in about 10 grains of sugar of milk can be divided after mixing it well. For convenience blank globules can be saturated with liquid medicines as already prescribed in that chapter and 2 globules for children and 4 for adults will make one dose.

In addition to medicines, some empty phials for making globules, some sugar of milk, and some blank globules should also be purchased. Powdered medicines, namely FERRUM PHOS. 6X, MAGNESIA PHOS. 6X, CALCAREA PHOS. 6X and KALI MUR. 6X, one ounce each, should also be purchased and kept separately. They are used usually in 5 grain doses with hot water. They are available in tablet form also but I prefer triturations (powders). Three mother tinctures of ARNICA, CALENDULA and CAMPHOR one ounce each should also be purchased and kept separately in another box. These medicines are now enough to treat ordinary ailments in one's family.

If you want to read more about Homoeopathy, *Organon of Medicine*, by Dr. Hahnemann himself is the best book. It is said to be the bible of Homoeopathy.

Kent's *Lectures on Homoeopathic Philosophy* is another book which deals with the philosophy of Homoeopathy in a masterly way.

To study individual drugs Dr. Demeys' *Essentials of Materia Medica* is a good handy book. For a detailed study Kent's *Lectures on Materia Medica* gives the best picture of a medicine.